KICK
SUGAR

Reawaken your taste buds
and boost your health

James Goolnik BDS MSc

Published in 2020 by Bow Lane Limited

Printed in Great Britain by Latitude Press Ltd

Photographer Rebecca Fennell
Editor Alice Sambrook
Designer Matt Inwood
Illustrator Jenny Dack

ISBN 978-1-5272-4941-7

A CIP catalogue record for this book is available from the British Library.

Text © James Goolnik, 2020
Photography © Rebecca Fennell, 2020

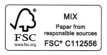

Cook's notes
• Recipes marked V are suitable for vegetarians and recipes marked V are suitable for vegans. In an effort to make this book as useful to as many people as possible, some of these recipes contain alternative ingredient options or serving suggestions which you should take care not to include if you wish to cater for vegetarians or vegans. An optional serving suggestion such as crème fraîche would not be suitable for vegans. There are some cheeses (such as Parmesan and Gruyère) which contain animal rennet and are not suitable for vegetarians, so you should swap these for a vegetarian alternative. Always check the food labels first and always read the recipe carefully.
• All eggs are medium unless otherwise specified.
• Always defrost frozen dishes overnight in the fridge before reheating thoroughly the next day.

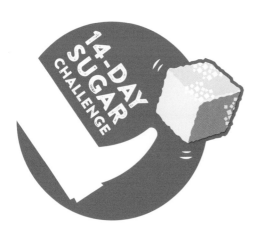

CONTENTS

FOREWORD
by chefs Katie and Giancarlo Caldesi

"Apple juice, no!" exclaimed James Goolnik.

It was our first visit to see him as our new family dentist. Giorgio, our son, was little and James was horrified to see he had a cavity. I told him that we had given him apple juice in a bottle at night to help him get off to sleep (I thought it was healthier than full-fat baby's milk). I had no idea that it would leave a sugary coating on his teeth for the night and cause irreversible damage.

I now know that sugar lurks in many forms and that it was responsible, not only for our children's tooth decay, but also for my husband's, Giancarlo's, type 2 diabetes. I have a lot of reasons to dislike it.

James came to our cookery school 16 years ago and we have been friends ever since. We are so impressed by his tireless work for his charity Rewards Project and it confirms that we are on the same crusade to inform everyone about how what we eat affects our health.

We have been friends with nutritionist Jenny Phillips since Giancarlo went to seek her help on reversing his diabetes. Jenny helped us to follow a low-carb diet and we became so inspired that together we wrote *The Diabetes Weight-loss Cookbook*, which offers a life-changing diet to reverse type 2 diabetes. The book shot to the bestsellers list, which demonstrates the strong public interest in avoiding sugar and carbs.

We have cut the sugar in the desserts in our restaurants, as we are aware that tastes are changing. Sugar is cheap and too many food manufacturers use it to pad out poor quality food. It is often used in low-fat food options such as fruit yoghurts, which people perceive to be healthy choices. We encourage people to consume natural, unprocessed foods and to read packaging labels carefully.

What we have found is that by using the natural sweetness of low-sugar fruits, such as berries and moderate amounts of apple, you can bring enough sweetness to popular recipes. Also, that using good quality vanilla extract and spices like cinnamon can make foods taste sweet even though they may not contain sugar.

Almost every household in Italy grows herbs on windowsills, outside their front door or in their gardens. Italians will also pick them from the wild. We love herbs, too, and we encourage the students at our cookery school to cook with them and garnish finished recipes with them. They look good, smell lovely and bring that all-important flavour to your dishes.

It isn't hard to cook from scratch. With a little planning, it soon becomes the natural way to live. The two weeks' worth of easy recipes in this book will give you a kick-start in the kitchen. Make the commitment to follow the two-week plan on your own, with friends or family. You have nothing to lose by trying!

If our family can come off sugar with a sugar-addict husband, two teenage and still-growing sons, a busy work life and being constantly surrounded by food in our restaurants, then anyone can do it! This book is for busy people like us, so you will find the recipes delicious, easy and quick to prepare. I want more people to discover that the key to good health is in what we eat. We have shown that you can reverse diabetes through diet, so why not start to change your own eating habits for the better and boost your health in as little as 14 days!

I'll leave the last word on this life-changing programme to my husband, Giancarlo:

"To be part of this book is very important to me, as I was a sugar addict for most of my life. I remember as a child never having enough Torrone (Italian nougat) and then feeling sick after polishing it all off. To be able to leave sugar behind is such an achievement and has transformed my health. This book will give you the start that you are looking for. If it can work for me, it will work for you."

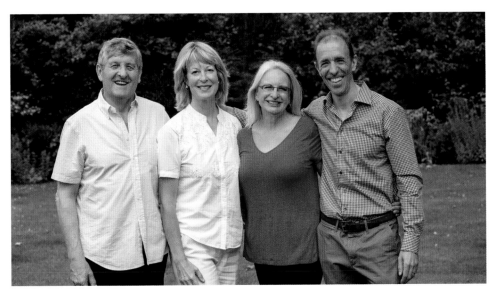

Giancarlo, Katie and Jenny with James

THE TEAM BEHIND THIS BOOK

This book would not have been possible without a great support team behind me. **Giancarlo and Katie Caldesi** provided the generous foreword above, but it was Giancarlo's advice and recipes which gave me the impetus for the dishes you'll find here in *Kick Sugar*, and it was Katie's knowledge that helped me to formulate them into a cookbook. Between them, they have so much knowledge and experience in the world of cheffing, writing and enjoying food and this book is all the richer for it.

Jenny Phillips is a science-based Nutritional Therapist. She helped me to truly understand what happens inside the body once you swallow sugar and she helped to co-write two of the chapters in this book. Her transition into nutrition was the result of her own journey of recovering from a cancer diagnosis in 2003. She published her first book *Eat to Outsmart Cancer* in 2015. Her second book *The Diabetes Weight-loss Cookbook* was co-authored with Giancarlo and Katie Caldesi and Dr David Unwin. Jenny is also a qualified yoga teacher and offers retreats and workshops. Her website is www.InspiredNutrition.co.uk.

INTRODUCTION

Welcome to your health boost! If you are looking to have more energy, not feel hungry all the time, get better sleep and have clearer skin, then this book is for you! By reading it, you are taking your first step towards educating and empowering yourself to break free of sugar.

Perhaps you have tried numerous "diets" in the past, but just ended up reaching for an easy way out? You will be relieved to hear that this is not another diet book, but an enjoyable and sustainable guide to healthy eating. In this book, we are going to show you how to cook with a beautiful array of real unprocessed foods – without the overdose of sugar.

One of the main barriers to healthy eating is a lack of knowledge about nutrition, so we are going to arm you with that knowledge and help you decipher the labels on food so that you can make informed choices when you shop. However, the ultimate aim of this meal plan is to get you cooking more food from scratch so that you don't need to spend all your time studying labels!

Research has found that after just six days of low sugar, your palate will recalibrate and you will start to notice how sweet normal foods/drinks taste.

What is the 14-Day Challenge?

As you will see, this is not a detox but a careful plan to gradually reduce your sugar intake over 14 days so that you can get back in control. That's right: just 14 days, with you following our team of experts, to help you kick sugar.

I have teamed up with one of our patrons, professional chef Giancarlo Caldesi, along with nutritionist Jenny Phillips and Clare Gray, a dietitian, to produce this cookbook. In these pages, you will find 14 days' worth of delicious recipes, along with help and information on how to retrain your palate. My team and I are going to help you understand your relationship with sugar and how to break free of it. This is not just a recipe book, it is a journey to reawakening your taste buds!

We'll explore how you can use other ingredients like herbs and spices to find remarkable flavour without the need for sugar. I am going to share with you the history of sugar and how it has become such a problem in our society. I will teach you about the different kinds of sugars, how to recognise them in shop-bought food, how much sugar is actually too much and what an excess of it does to your body (in terms of appearance, physical and mental health). I want to help you understand your relationship with sugar and give you some strategies to help you cope without it. There is a chapter on preparation for the 14-day challenge and a list of kitchen essentials, with help and advice on how to stock up your cupboards. We will also look at whether you currently reward yourself and your family with sugar, and how to combat this.

So, why has a dentist set up a charity and what has it got to do with this cookbook?

Do you know the number one reason for a five-year-old being admitted to hospital in the UK? Actually, I will make it easier for you, it is the same for six, seven, eight and nine-year-olds.

Yes, tooth decay! Shocking isn't it? Especially when it is entirely preventable. Tooth decay is the most common disease affecting children (Marshall et al 2003) and it is 100% down to diet. Having decayed teeth affects speech, nutrition, growth, eating and social interactions.

Being a dentist, I am spending more and more of my time repairing the damage sugar has done. Dentists are losing the battle against sugar, there is just as much tooth decay as there was when I first qualified. Despite the advances in modern medicine and almost universal use of fluoride toothpaste in the UK, tooth decay is on the rise. Enamel is the hardest substance in our bodies, but once destroyed it does not grow back. It is attacked by acid which is a by-product of all the sugar we eat. Tooth decay is an early warning sign that there is too much sugar in your diet.

Over my 26 years in dental practice, my team and I have been guiding our patients at Bow Lane Dental Group to replace the sugar in their diets. Not only do their teeth and mouths become healthier but also the rest of their bodies. There is a clear link between obesity and oral health. Most people see their dental teams more often than their doctor so this gives us a unique opportunity to help. I talk to all my patients about diet and exercise and gently nudge them by giving them tips on snacking, different exercises or meditation apps. On a weekly basis, my team and I spot the signs of other disease by subtle changes in our patients' mouths. In the majority of cases, these people are unaware of any problems and we refer them to the relevant specialists before it is too late.

With a busy job and a family with three children myself, I am aware of the time pressures involved with keeping everyone fuelled throughout the day. We still have birthday cakes and desserts in our family, but we believe that sugar is not for every day. We are aware of when we are eating it and, as our ancestors did, we use it for celebrations. I get angry when manufacturers add sugar to nearly everything just because it is cheap and makes bad food taste palatable. Their objective is for us to buy more and eat more.

As a parent, I am fed up with fending off the sugar pushed to my children. At two years old, my youngest daughter was so excited to have her first haircut. At the end, what do you think the hairdresser got out? Yes, a huge jar of lollipops as a "reward" for her first haircut. This is wrong! She loved her first haircut anyway, and wouldn't it have been better to have a certificate that she could treasure and put on her wall rather than a two-minute sugar rush never to be thought about again?

When it's a child's birthday at school, they all bring in cakes – that can be over 20 birthdays a year! If you come top in a test, the reward is a chocolate bar. If you get an injection at the doctor, you get a sugar cube. When my 16-year-old daughter wanted to fundraise for her school, they chose to sell doughnuts. The doughnut company even has special rates for fundraising doughnuts.

I bet you all know lots of sugar pushers!

Sugar is so universally appealing and intertwined in our society, it is the easy, default answer. Everyone wants recognition because it is a great motivator, but it doesn't need to come from food or sugar. There must be a better way....

I decided it was time for change, so I put together a team of dentists, doctors, nutritionists, dietitians and psychologists to set up a charity called Rewards Project. We aim to transform the way we reward our children, so that this behaviour is not then modelled into adulthood. We are currently working with over 550 schools and nurseries looking at how they currently reward their children and helping them shift the rewards culture away from food and sugar. The first step was a review (the rewards review) to see where in the school day the children came into contact with sugar and, as you will read later, the results were astonishing. You can get involved by sending this rewards review to your children's schools or nurseries to see how we can help them.

Every day, my team and I help people get healthier by changing their diets. This cookbook will hopefully help thousands more people reduce their sugar intake and reboot their taste buds in order to experience a full range of tastes, rather than just sweet!

So, let's get started.

#ThinkBeyondSugar

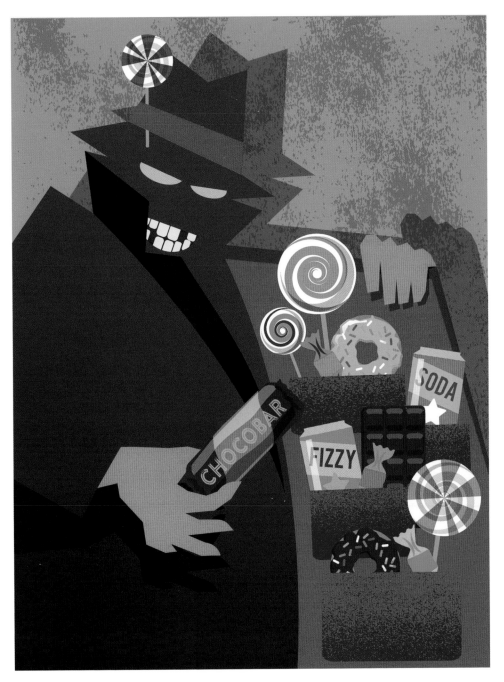

Do you know a sugar pusher? You may remember one from your childhood.

Monitoring your progress

Imagine if you woke before the alarm, feeling refreshed and raring to go? And then you had great energy throughout the day and slept like a baby at night? Is that even possible?

Yes, it is!

Jenny said *"I changed my eating habits, by cutting down on sugar, 16 years ago to help me survive through cancer treatment. But I hadn't banked on the many side effects – great energy, not feeling hungry all the time, better sleep, clear skin, improved digestion, less allergies (I was able to stop inhalers for asthma that I'd been taking since I was eight years old) and more."*

As this is a challenge, we need to set some parameters so that you can monitor your achievements and notice how your body and feelings change over the 14 days. We have developed a scorecard questionnaire that you should complete before you start the challenge, and then repeat at the end (see opposite).

Rate each statement between 1 (strongly agree) to 5 (strongly disagree). Circle the number that best represents how you feel. As all of these statements are in the positive, the lower your overall score, the better. There is also space here to include any health concerns that are individual to you. We will repeat this scorecard at the end of the book to encourage you to assess your improvements after following the 14-day sugar challenge.

Also, before you start the challenge, please also complete a three-day food and feelings diary, eating and drinking as you normally would (see pages 14–15). This will help you understand your relationship with food to begin with. We tend to underestimate what we eat and forget the grazing during the day. Also, it will be interesting to note your emotional state at the same time. Are you just eating because you are bored or stressed or is it because it is actually mealtime and you are hungry? People who complete this diary are much more likely to succeed in this challenge and ultimately change their eating behaviour.

All of our charts are available to print online at **www.rewardsproject.org** if you prefer not to write in this beautiful book.

TOP TIPS

Spend a moment to think about **WHY** you are doing this challenge to give you greater motivation. Is it for more energy? To sleep better? Lose weight? Have you had a health scare? Want to reduce your dental bills and keep your teeth for life?

The 14-Day Sugar Challenge
Questionnaire
Circle a number for each question

DATE					

DENTAL	Yes		No		
I saw my dentist in the last year					
I have no cavities/fillings					
My gums do not bleed when I brush					

SLEEP	Agree				Disagree
I sleep well at night	1	2	3	4	5
I wake feeling refreshed	1	2	3	4	5

MOOD	Agree				Disagree
I feel confident and happy	1	2	3	4	5

ENERGY	Agree				Disagree
I do not frequently feel tired	1	2	3	4	5
My energy does not slump in the day	1	2	3	4	5

WEIGHT	Agree				Disagree
I am happy with my weight	1	2	3	4	5

FOOD	Agree				Disagree
I enjoy my meals	1	2	3	4	5
I do not crave sweet or savoury foods	1	2	3	4	5
I am motivated to cook	1	2	3	4	5

HEALTH

Please add any concerns/issues such as joints, allergies, digestion etc.

Three-Day Food Diary

Record everything that you eat and drink over three days.
Try to make sure that at least one of those is a weekend day.

Remember to record:

➤ Everything you eat and drink
➤ The time at which you ate and how hungry you were feeling before you ate and your mood (e.g. bored)
➤ The number of teaspoons of sugar added to your food or drink

If it helps, carry the record with you and fill in the details as you go about your day – otherwise you are likely to forget. The more accurate the diary, the more likely you are to succeed in improving your behaviour.

If you prefer not to write in this beautiful book, all of our charts are available to print online at **www.rewardsproject.org**

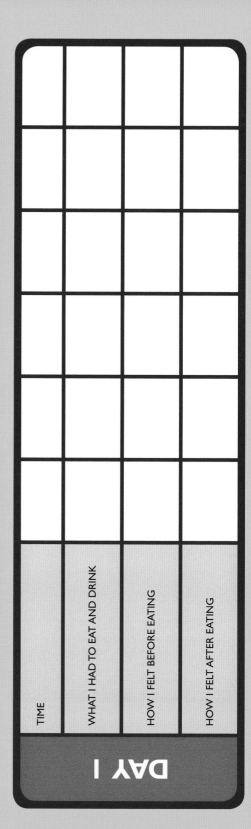

DAY 1							
TIME							
WHAT I HAD TO EAT AND DRINK							
HOW I FELT BEFORE EATING							
HOW I FELT AFTER EATING							

DAY 2

TIME						
WHAT I HAD TO EAT AND DRINK						
HOW I FELT BEFORE EATING						
HOW I FELT AFTER EATING						

DAY 3

TIME						
WHAT I HAD TO EAT AND DRINK						
HOW I FELT BEFORE EATING						
HOW I FELT AFTER EATING						

A HISTORY
OF SUGAR
AND JOY

In our caveman days, sweet treats were few and far between. They came only from fruits like berries, which we had to search for and were only available seasonally. Fast forward to just a few generations ago, and sugar was readily available as an ingredient. Grandma may have purchased it to make delicious cakes or biscuits, but this was only for high days and holidays, celebrations, special occasions or maybe to enjoy with the company of family and friends. Move on to the 21st century and we are surrounded by sweet foods everywhere, readily accessible, available and affordable almost 24/7. And it's not just the obvious drinks, cakes and sweets – many savoury products are also affected. A whopping 74% of food and beverage products in our grocery stores contain added sugars.

TOP TIPS

Visit www.sugarquiz.org to see how much sugar you and your children are consuming. You will receive a free report with tips on how you can cut down.

It is difficult to say no when everyone around you is eating junk food. Look into the typical dentist's or doctor's staff kitchen and it will be full of sugar and processed food. Why do even health professionals find it hard to say no when they know directly the consequences? If your tooth developed a cavity and started to hurt the moment you ate a biscuit, you would soon stop eating biscuits. The problem is that any negative effects from your diet take months or even years to materialise in your body. This delay allows us to dismiss the thought and say to ourselves it won't happen to me.

Chances are, if you've picked up this book you are joining the many of us who are re-examining our relationship with the sweet stuff. Welcome aboard!

I think it best we start at the beginning and look at where our obsession with sugar comes from, what it does to our bodies and why we use it to reward ourselves.

The timeline of sugar

Before sugar, honey was the most prevalent sweetening agent. It was used in religious ceremonies (and still is today in some cultures), to make medicines more palatable, to spice food and to ferment into alcohol (mead). The first reference to sugar was around 286 BC in China. It was first brought to Europe from India by the returning troops of Alexander the Great, but it wasn't until over a thousand years later, after the end of the Crusades, that this "sweet salt" would start to have an impact on us.

In the late 15th century, the discovery of the New World brought the sugar cane plant to Europe. Sugar eventually took over from honey as the preferred sweetener because of its more neutral taste. Originally used as a spice and for decoration, it was a privilege enjoyed only by the wealthy due to its huge cost. Sugar was too expensive for commoners meaning they were better at keeping their teeth free from decay. It slowly became woven into the rituals of society, served as the sweet end to a meal and to celebrate a life event or festival.

In the 16th century, a French agronomist discovered that sugar could also be made from the sugar beet plant and sugar plantations became more widespread. Dentists started noticing that sugar caused teeth to rot, prompting a backlash against sugar and making it fall out of favour with the rich and powerful; but this didn't stop it from moving down the social chain. In the skulls from the London plague pits of 1665, they found large amounts of dental disease. There had been a rise in tea drinking, as a result of the claims of its health benefits, and as the cost came down, hot tea sweetened with sugar was widely drunk by working-class people.

In the 18th Century, the vast spread of the sugar plantations and the industrial revolution reduced the cost of refined sugar further. More and more people had access to sugar, and it became known as the "opiate of the people". Tobacco, sugar and tea were some of the first products to become cultural symbols of sophistication. The general population could pretend to be upper class with their cup of sweetened tea because of its lingering associations with wealth. By 1840, sweet manufacturers discovered mass production of hard sweets so that more people could indulge. In 1885, John Pemberton developed Coca-Cola as a headache and hangover remedy. His original recipe contained cocaine – in the form of an extract of the coca leaf, which inspired the "Coca" part of the name. The current recipe is still a secret, but cocaine has since been removed. Food manufacturers worked out that the more sugar they put in, the better their food seemed to taste and the more addictive it seemed to be. Furthermore, they discovered that the preservative effects of sugar would increase the shelf-life of products and thus further increase their profits.

Sugar has no nutritional benefit and the food manufacturers purely put it in to boost their sales!

Not only does having too much sugar make some people sick, it also leaves them needing medication, which then drives up the pharmaceutical industry's profits. So, it is not in the food or pharmaceutical companies' interests to cut out the sugar, but it is in the interest of our health!

In 2019, researchers from Queen Mary University of London looked at the skulls of 224 adults, predominantly from the 17th century, examining a total of 5,195 teeth and compared them to modern-day Londoners. They were shocked to discover our 17th-century predecessors had fewer missing teeth and less decay. Despite the lack of dental care in post-medieval times, they had better teeth than we do now.

TOP TIPS

Sweetness is even in toothpaste. Take a look at your tube and you will almost certainly find saccharin or the sugar alcohols sorbitol or xylitol. In this challenge, we want you to use a toothpaste without sweeteners. We don't want to start the day stimulating all your sweet receptors! The Kick Sugar team have developed the world's first toothpaste with Fluoride and NO sweeteners. See our website for more details.

Why sugar makes us happy

Why is it that the sweet taste of sugar is so appealing? Most of us now know sugar is bad for us. It causes illnesses and shortens our lives. So why do we still eat it? To understand this, we need to talk about the brain and biochemistry.

It is our hormones that drive our behaviour.

Eating sugar causes dopamine to be released, which is the chemical of rewards. It leads our drive for food and sex, and it has helped humans survive for so many years. You may recognise this as that 'ahh' moment when you first take a bite of something sugary. In fact, this is primed in us from birth when the sweetness of breast milk both soothes us and encourages us to suckle. Scientists have even shown how a four-month old human foetus can respond to sweetness in amniotic fluid by swallowing more.

In today's overstimulated world, our dopamine levels are all over the place with many people addicted to short-term dopamine boosts. Have you noticed what you do as soon as you get bored at work or on a task at home? Rather than struggling through or taking a break, most people distract themselves by checking their phone, emails, social media or eating something sweet. All of which releases dopamine.

The problem is that with prolonged exposure to stimulants like sugar, the signal gets weaker. Thus, you have to consume more sugar for your body to get the same hit of dopamine because your tolerance levels are increased. Hence the reason for addictions to foods, drugs, smoking and alcohol, plus behaviours such as gambling, shopping and sex.

If we are talking about stress, we need also to talk about the neurotransmitter serotonin, manufactured by our bodies from the amino acid, tryptophan. Serotonin is believed to help regulate mood, appetite, digestion, sleep and sexual desire and function. Deficiency of it is thought to cause clinical depression. Low levels have been found to increase our craving for sweet or starchy foods. Drug companies are happy to sell us drugs to increase our serotonin levels, but you can also help with what you eat. Steering clear of sugar helps, as does consuming foods rich in tryptophan like egg yolks, cheese, turkey and nuts. Exercising also triggers the release of tryptophan into your blood, as does sunlight.

When we are stressed, the hormone cortisol is released, which often causes us to increase our food intake, especially of high sugar foods. If this stress becomes chronic, then food can become an addiction. People describe the symptoms of withdrawal when they suddenly deprive themselves of sugar-rich foods. In some circumstances, excessive sugar intake can lead to behavioural (bingeing, withdrawal and craving) and neurochemical changes identical to those in drug addiction.

Once we are addicted to one substance, it is much easier for our bodies to become addicted to others. This is because our dopamine receptors are less reactive; this is called the gateway theory. This challenge will help you get off sugar so you will be less likely to become addicted to others or make it easier for you to get off others. It will also allow your dopamine receptors to take a rest and reboot, leading to a lifting of your energy level and stabilising your mood.

FALSE BELIEFS

• **STRESS IS BAD**
Your body needs stress to function. Think of the fight-or-flight response. What we do not need is stress that stays around for weeks or months. It can weaken the immune system and cause high blood pressure, fatigue, depression, anxiety and even heart disease.

• **WE ARE NOW EATING LESS SUGAR**
Over the past 300 years sugar consumption in the UK has actually increased from 1.8kg to 23kg per person per year, with low-income groups now consuming the most.

Opposite: the effect that processed food and sugar can have on the stress cycle

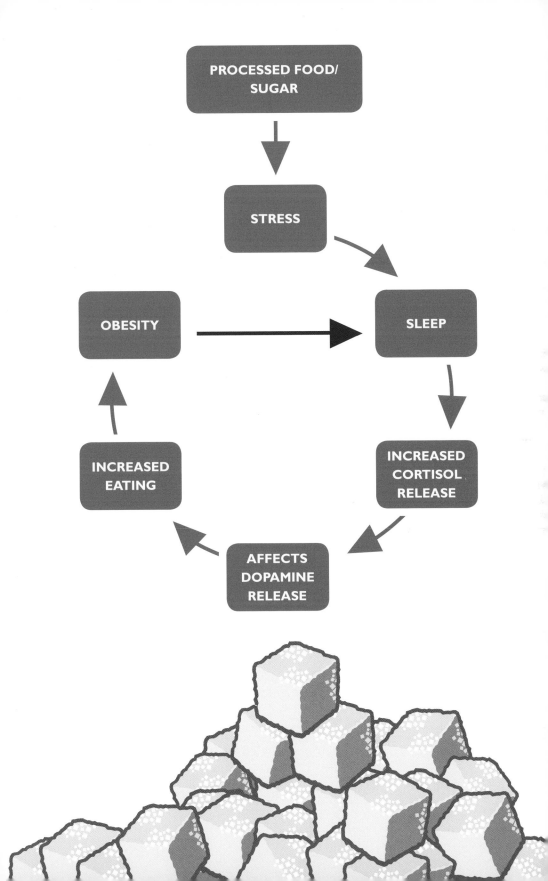

2

SUGAR
AND OUR
BODIES

co-written with Nutritional Therapist, Jenny Phillips

What is sugar?

The term "sugar" commonly refers to what we know as table sugar, the stuff we use in baking and that some people add to their tea and coffee. But as we will cover in this book, sugar comes in many other forms and goes by many additional names. The more we break this down for you, the more you will be able to recognise it when you see it. Sugars are part of the food group known as carbohydrates (or carbs). There are three types of carbohydrates:

1. Starches or complex carbohydrates

These contain long strings of glucose molecules, a type of sugar, which when found in potatoes, vegetables and whole grains like oats and wheat can be a good source of energy. These are often described as "good carbs" because they release their sugars slowly. But beware of refined or ultra-processed foods like biscuits and crackers as these release their glucose molecules very quickly and are therefore associated with similar health issues to regular sugar.

Any food made from wheat, rice, oats, cornmeal, barley or another cereal grain is a grain product which contains starches. This includes bread, pasta and breakfast cereals. Grains can be further divided into whole or refined.

Whole grains These contain the entire grain kernel – the bran, germ, and endosperm e.g. wholemeal flour, bulgur (cracked wheat) and brown rice.

Refined grains These have been milled, a process that removes the bran and germ. This gives grains a finer texture and improves their shelf life, but removes dietary fibre, iron, and many B vitamins e.g. white flour, white bread and white rice. Some manufacturers try and get around this by adding vitamins back in after processing (enriched grains), but this doesn't have the same effect. Since the fibre has been stripped from enriched grains (and not re-added), these processed foods will not keep your blood sugar levels steady. **We recommend you only eat whole grains** rather than refined grains during this challenge as they are so much better for you, see page 74 for a list.

Whole grains have complex carbohydrates which give bacteria less digestible food for them to grow. Plus, they offer plenty of other nutrients that actively help your teeth and gums to stay healthy.

Good carbs Anything using whole grains like wholemeal bread, oats, brown rice, wholemeal pasta and all types of vegetables.

Bad carbs Anything using refined grains like white flour, or ultra-processed foods such as biscuits, chocolates, sweets, chicken nuggets, energy bars and carbonated and sugared sweet drinks.

If you are pre-diabetic or diagnosed with diabetes, then you may want to reduce your intake of starchy carbohydrates even more than in this plan, as you will not tolerate carbohydrates well. Please discuss any diet changes with a medical professional first.

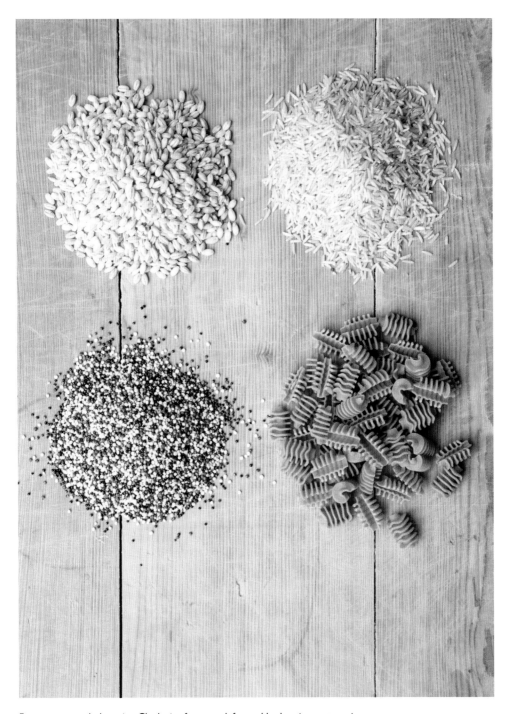

Four common whole grains. Clockwise from top-left: pearl barley, rice, pasta, quinoa

2. Sugars

This includes both added sugar and natural sugars found in things like milk and fruit. The most common sugar is sucrose, a di-saccharide – or two molecules of simple carbohydrates joined together. These molecules are glucose and fructose. Glucose is the molecule which your body uses to make energy; fructose gives foods their sweet taste and can only be processed by liver cells, which convert it into fat. Fructose is not needed by the body to survive.

The sugar content of a food is usually shown on the label below the carbohydrate content. There are two types – free sugar, which is the added sugar, or natural sugars which are contained within things like fruit or milk. Your body doesn't differentiate between the two and will respond to both in exactly the same way by releasing glucose into the bloodstream.

People often say that milk is good for teeth because of the calcium content. It's true that it is an important source of calcium and phosphorus and it also contains the protein casein, which helps to protect teeth from acids in the mouth. It does contain lactose, which at low levels does not lead to tooth decay. We advise, though, that children should not be put to bed with a bottle containing milk, just water.

3. Fibre

The third type of carbohydrate, fibre, is the indigestible portion of our food that feeds our gut microbes and is helpful for good gut health. Fibre helps to slow down the absorption of sugar, which is why it is preferable to eat a whole piece of fruit rather than just drink fruit juice. Fruit is changed when it gets juiced, almost all of the fibrous material gets removed. This is why you can rightly only manage to eat one or two apples in one afternoon, but you could quite easily drink a litre of apple juice. The pulp, skin and fibre fill you up and limit your consumption. Foods high in fibre require more chewing, which increases your saliva production, therefore more harmful bacteria are removed from your mouth when you eat them.

Now you understand carbs and having balance in your meals. You will see in the recipe section the nutritional information for each meal is clearly laid out. For growth and development your body requires carbs, fats and proteins. Fat is a source of essential fatty acids, which the body cannot make itself. They help the body absorb vitamins A, D, E and K plus keep your skin and hair healthy. Protein helps make you feel full and has the highest thermic effect, meaning it takes more calories to digest compared to carbs or fats. You will see in our recipes lots of sources of protein. Look for lean animal-based sources like meat, fish, poultry, eggs and dairy. Protein is also from plant-based sources like soy, grains and certain vegetables.

How much is too much sugar?

There are two main concerns about the prevalence of added sugars in our foods. Firstly, there is the "crowding out" issue, where sweet foods replace more nutritious foods as a source of calories. Once someone has developed a taste for sugar, this may directly discourage them from eating other foods that don't give that same intensely sweet "hit". This reduces our appreciation for the many other tastes and flavours that the world has to offer. In this challenge, we want to open all those options up again for you.

Secondly, sweet foods are high in calories and extremely easy to overindulge in, fuelling a calorific excess which is apparent not only in our growing waistlines, but also in the rise of diet-related diseases.

Chronic health conditions related to diet:

Cardiovascular (heart) disease
Hypertension (high blood pressure)
Type 2 diabetes
Strokes
Some cancers

Because of these issues, the World Health Organisation (WHO) and Public Health England have recently lowered recommended sugar intake levels. Both organisations state that added sugars should be kept below 5% of total calories, although some guidelines (such as in the US) still state 10%.

Eating sugar is not essential for life because our body can make energy from a wide range of non-sugary foods, so there is no need to eat it. So why are sugars advised at all? Dr Priyanka Wali gave a powerful speech at the USDA 2020 Dietary Guidelines asking to change the excess sugar limit recommendation from 10% to zero. She also proposed a reduced recommended carb intake by half to reflect the current health status of many citizens.

We agree. However, that doesn't mean that you cannot enjoy the odd treat on special occasions and holidays if you are otherwise healthy. But eating sweet foods every day will likely be a disaster for your long-term health, especially if you have prediabetes or diabetes (which up to half of the developed world has). This challenge will help you to take out much of the added sugar in your diet. After the challenge, you can then choose how and when you replace it, if at all.

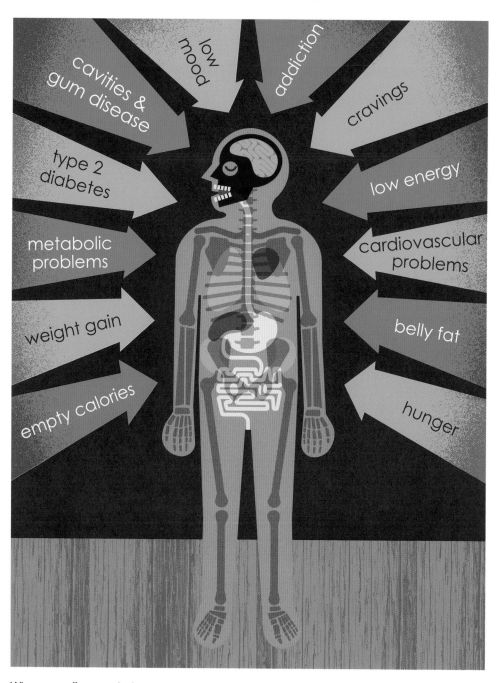

Where sugar affects your body

The effects of sugar

Low mood
sugar can affect how you feel

Addiction
sugar acts like a drug, flooding your brain with dopamine

Cardiovascular disease
sugar raises blood pressure and increases blood fats (triglycerides)

Cavities and gum disease
it feeds bacteria in your mouth, which damages gums and tooth enamel

Metabolic problems
sugar causes insulin resistance, which can lead to diabetes

Type 2 diabetes
sugar from both sweet and starchy foods causes diabetes

Skin
it increases both inflammation in your body and oil production leading to acne and ageing of your skin

Weight gain
sugar is converted into body fat in the liver

Belly fat
even skinny people may have a tum, courtesy of insulin

Hunger
sugar causes you to be resistant to the hormone leptin, so you don't feel full

Cravings
it can make you obsess about food

Empty calories
sugar doesn't contain any nutrients

Low energy
sugar drops your energy like a stone in as little as 30 minutes

There are so many health problems associated with sugar overload. These may be part of the reason that you are looking to cut down, or you may not be aware that some of these are caused by sugar at all. I will expand on four of the most important effects in the pages that follow – dental health, diabetes, weight gain and mental health.

Sugar and dental health

For the past 26 years, I have been repairing the damage sugar does to teeth. Dental enamel is the hardest substance in our bodies, but it gets dissolved by dental decay (caries), which is the world's most prevalent bacterial infection.

We all have millions of bacteria in our bodies, most of which are vital for our health. However, some of these bacteria cause tooth decay and gum disease, the most common being Streptococcus mutans. These bacteria in your mouth react with certain foods to produce acid. This acidic environment is created within just 3–5 minutes of eating and does not recover for 45–60 minutes (Rugg-Gunn and Nunn 1999).

For decay to happen you need four things:

1. **Sugar** Without free (added) sugar your teeth do not decay – period!
2. **Decay-producing bacteria in the mouth** Not everyone has these. That is why some people can eat a lot of sugary things and their teeth do not rot. However, other parts of their body will suffer instead, like the liver.
3. **Teeth** Without teeth then the bacteria have nothing to attack.
4. **Time** It takes a minimum of three months for teeth to decay.

Think of dental decay as an early warning sign that your diet needs correcting. Whilst sugar is the number one criminal, starches are also a source of carbohydrate that can cause tooth decay, especially if cooked. Starches on their own are low risk to teeth (pasta, for example) but eaten in combination with sugar will turbocharge the speed at which your teeth will decay (Duarte et al 2008) due to changing the environment for the bacteria to flourish (biofilm). Once the bacteria overstay their welcome, they join together and create a sticky build-up or plaque that sticks to your teeth and is harder to remove.

When you eat a sugar/starch combination (e.g. biscuits) as a snack, this has an even worse effect on teeth than when consumed as part of a meal for two reasons. The first is because the bacteria in your mouth have a steady supply of food and keep producing acid, so your teeth are constantly bathed in acid. Your saliva just cannot keep up! The second is, this combination of food sticks even harder to your teeth, and without eating other fibrous foods then stays there until your next meal or when it is time to brush your teeth before bed.

> "Tooth decay is a continual process with alternating periods of demineralisation and remineralisation." (Silverstone 1977)

So how can you reduce your chance of getting caries? Well, the number one factor is diet – reduce your frequency and amount of eating and drinking sugar and carbohydrates. We thought initially it was all about reducing frequency of sugar intake, but new research shows the total amount of free sugars is more important. Our aim in this book is to reduce the total amounts of sugars consumed by working on frequency first to help reduce the total amount consumed.

Other factors can slow down the progression of caries, such as brushing and flossing, but your teeth will still decay. It is a false belief that you can eat what you want and as long as you brush afterwards you will not get decay. It will slow the process down, as will using a fluoride mouth rinse, but it cannot stop it. This book will show that, by simply changing your diet, you have the power to stop decay forever. Not only will you be saving money, you will make dental visits more pleasant. I do not want to drill your teeth as much as you don't want me to drill them!

Talking about brushing, most people do not brush correctly. Why is this? Probably because we were never taught so we just copy our parents or copy what we see on the screen. Characters in programmes

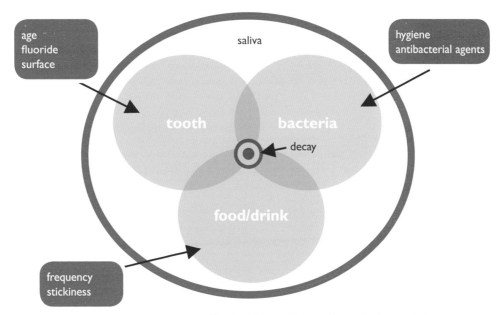

age
fluoride
surface

saliva

hygiene
antibacterial agents

tooth

bacteria

← decay

food/drink

frequency
stickiness

The three factors which combine to lead to tooth decay over time

are often brushing their teeth whilst doing something else with lots of foam coming out of their mouths! What is the purpose of tooth brushing? To remove the majority of the food and bacteria around your teeth without damaging your teeth or gums. I often get asked what is the best brush. Firstly, you can do just as good a job with a manual brush, but make sure you choose a brush head that is not too big; a medium or size 35 is ideal for most adults. If you prefer an electric toothbrush, choose one with a small head and crucially a timer. We recommend brushing for 2 minutes so having a timer helps with this. Please just brush your teeth and don't try and check your phone at the same time. At least once per week look in the mirror and check you are cleaning where the teeth meet the gums.

Start by placing your manual toothbrush at a 45-degree angle to the gums. Gently move the brush back and forth in short strokes (covering 1–2 teeth at a time maximum). For electric brushes use the same angle. Remember, scrubbing away with your electric toothbrush is not necessary – instead it is simply a matter of holding it in place for a few seconds before moving along to the next tooth.

It is best to brush in the same order each time so as not to miss bits. Brush the outer surfaces then the inner surfaces, and finish with the chewing surfaces of the teeth. Disclosing tablets (vegetable dyes that stain the plaque in your mouth) are a good idea to use once per week to help show you any areas that you may have missed.

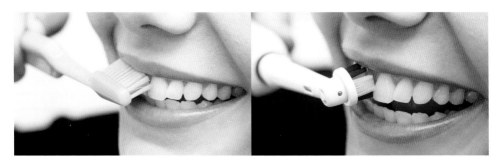

Note the angle of the toothbrush

Flossing – do you need to do it?

Well if you want to live six years longer! In his book *The Real Age Makeover*, Dr. Michael Roizen showed that on average you will live 6.4 years longer if you floss regularly. This is because no matter how brilliant your brushing technique, you cannot remove the plaque between your teeth. This plaque builds up over the day, then turns into tartar, a hard deposit that can irritate and inflame the gums. This tartar and inflammation can cause the gums to recede and create a gap between the gum and the tooth (a pocket) that could become infected. This stage is called periodontal disease, which has been linked heart disease, HPV infection, mouth cancers, diabetes and kidney failure. This is where flossing or the use of interdental brushes comes in. It removes this plaque preventing gum disease in the first place. You do need to remove this once per day to stop it building up.

Most people cannot keep their mouths clean enough to prevent dental decay without professional dental help, such as visiting the dental hygienist. Decay usually starts in inaccessible locations like in-between teeth or in deep grooves on the biting surfaces. Your dentist can easily fill these grooves by applying what's called a "fissure sealant".

The most common age for getting dental decay is in childhood. As you get older, usually your diet improves and you take better care of your teeth. It then gets worse in the elderly as their saliva is less capable of preventing decay and their gums recede, exposing the root surface of the teeth, which are less resistant to acids.

Why are my teeth sensitive?

More and more people are experiencing sensitive teeth. This is down to a combination of diet and us keeping our teeth for longer. As I mentioned earlier, the enamel on our teeth protects them from the harsh environment of the mouth. If this enamel is worn down from grinding (bruxism), over-brushing or acid, the roots or dentine is exposed. This dentine has thousands of pores (tubules) that connect to the nerve (pulp) of your tooth. Inside these tubules there are tiny cells called odontoblasts which help protect and repair our teeth from decay. Normally these tubules are blocked but they can easily be opened by overbrushing and acids in our diet. The first signs are your tooth is sensitive to sweet/sour or temperature. This is why after a night of drinking alcohol your teeth can be very sensitive, the tubules have been opened by the acid. They can be either physically blocked by toothpastes or your dentist can apply gels or varnishes to reduce the excitability of these odontoblasts.

Sensitive toothpaste can help block these tubules but it often requires regular application over a week period before they are sufficiently blocked and then can easily be reopened if you stop using the toothpaste or have another acid attack.

If your teeth continue to be sensitive after a week, please do make an appointment to see your dentist as it may be a sign of something else.

Toothpastes

We talk a lot about reading the labels on packaging in this challenge and the number one ingredient to look out for in a toothpaste is fluoride. Fluoride is a naturally occurring mineral found in water and certain foods such as black tea. Around 10% of the population of the United Kingdom receives fluoridated water. It was first proven over 100 years ago to help strengthen teeth and it is still our first defence against decay. It is incorporated into the enamel to strengthen it and make it more resistant to the acid attacks in your mouth. Regular applications of fluoride are needed to keep this enamel resistance;

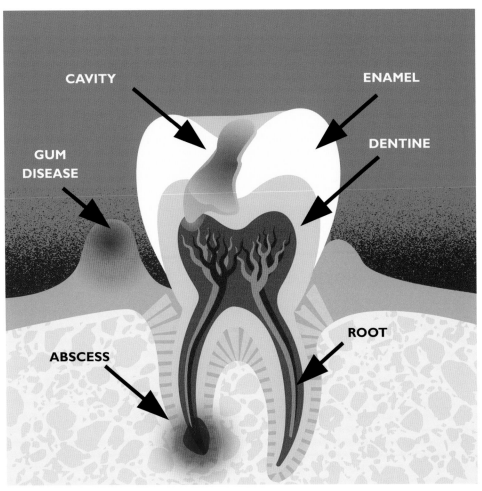

A molar tooth

hence you should use it for life if you want healthy teeth. Children should use a fluoride toothpaste 1,000 parts per million (ppm) up until aged two. Above age three a fluoride level of 1,350–1,500ppm should be used. Once they get adult teeth (usually from age six), they can start using adult toothpaste (around 1500 ppm fluoride). The rest of the toothpaste ingredients are largely put in for stain removal and to make it taste nice. One ingredient to try and avoid is SLS (Sodium Lauryl Sulphate). It is a foaming agent that makes some people more prone to mouth ulcers and has no health benefit. Check out the Kick Sugar Fluoride toothpaste with no sweeteners or SLS and it tastes great with the herbs mint and cinnamon.

Mouthwashes

As a general rule, us dentists do not recommend mouthwash. There has been some evidence to suggest that regular use of alcohol-containing rinses increases your risk of mouth cancer. If you have a sore mouth, ulcer or have had some mouth surgery, the gold standard remedy is salty water, as salt is a natural disinfectant. 1 tablespoon of salt should be dissolved in a glass of warm water and gargled for 30 seconds 2–3 times a day for up to three weeks. If you are going to use a mouthwash, make sure it is an alcohol-free one and think of it as a type of mouth deodoriser like a perfume or aftershave.

If you don't like the taste of artificial mouthwashes, then try this recipe: Mix 1 part pure unsweetened aloe vera juice, to 4 parts of water, 2 teaspoons bicarbonate of soda (optional) and add 2 drops of peppermint essential oil for taste. Just use as a mouthwash, don't swallow.

Sugars and gum disease

A high frequency of consumption of added sugars will increase your body's inflammation in relation to gum disease. We know that gum disease in diabetic patients is more aggressive, leading to faster breakdown of their gums and the bones around their teeth, eventually resulting in tooth loss. We also know that the chronic inflammation in gum disease actually contributes to further diabetic complications. Someone with diabetes needs to clean their teeth more thoroughly and see their hygienist and dentist more regularly. This will not only prevent gum problems, but will also stop complications in the rest of their body.

Sugar and diabetes

Rates of diabetes have doubled since the 1980s and the WHO estimates that this chronic and potentially crippling disease now affects over 422 million people worldwide. If you don't suffer with it yourself, it is likely that you'll know someone who does.

There are two types of diabetes – type 1 and type 2. The latter is the most prevalent, accounting for 90% of cases, and is strongly linked with diet and lifestyle choices. However, people with type 1 diabetes will also benefit from the recipes here. (If you are taking medication, then please discuss any diet changes with your medical professional.)

Diabetes is diagnosed when glucose, which comes from both the starchy and sugary foods we consume, rises in the blood stream. Glucose is used for making energy, but an overload of it causes problems in the body in both the short and the longer term.

Blood glucose levels are usually tightly controlled by the body – too low (hypoglycaemia) is a dangerous state which can lead to unconsciousness or worse. Too high (hyperglycaemia) and the sugar itself can wreak untold damage on the body. This is why diabetes has such devastating effects if not controlled through diet and medication (if required). It may surprise you to learn that there are less than two teaspoons of glucose in your blood stream, which explains why regular sugar surges from foods and drinks are so problematic. Your can of cola contains around nine teaspoons of sugar.

The amount of glucose in the blood stream is controlled by one master hormone – insulin. This important hormone shuttles the glucose into cells to make energy and takes any excess to the liver.

Here's what should happen:

- You EAT foods containing sugar (glucose and fructose) and/or starchy foods (strings of glucose)
- They are DIGESTED to release glucose into the blood and, consequently, blood levels rise
- It is CONTROLLED by releasing insulin which returns blood glucose levels back to normal

However, problems arise when insulin is either insufficient (type 1 or later type 2) or the insulin doesn't work properly (type 2). This is called insulin resistance and refers to when glucose levels fail to normalise, even when insulin levels are really high. The result in both cases is that glucose levels in the blood stream remain too high.

Cutting down on sugary foods and beverages is the most obvious way to reduce your risk of getting diabetes. You are reducing the amount of glucose that your body is exposed to. One study using data from 175 countries showed that just one can of sweet soda per day leads to a dramatic increase in the rate of diabetes. A further study estimates that **regular consumption of sugar-sweetened beverages (1–2 per day) increases diabetes risk by 26%.**

In addition, the fructose part of sugary foods and drinks can have a detrimental effect on liver function, potentially contributing to fatty liver disease. When teenage children with metabolic syndrome (see below) were subjected to a diet change which removed all sugar containing foods and beverages, their health markers (including insulin sensitivity) significantly improved, confirming that fructose does play a role in the development of diabetes.

If you have already been diagnosed with prediabetes or diabetes, then you could consider restricting both sugar and also starchy foods, like bread, pasta and rice, which break down to sugar.

25% of adults in the UK suffer from metabolic syndrome. It is a diagnosis when someone has three or more of the following risk factors:

- high blood pressure
- insulin resistance – where the hormone insulin is less able to keep the amount of sugar in the blood at a healthy level
- obesity – especially around the waistline
- unhealthy levels of blood fats – usually high triglyceride levels and low HDL levels

On their own they can damage blood vessels and organs, but combined they are particularly dangerous and can increase the risk of type 2 diabetes, heart attacks or strokes.

Sugar and weight gain

Of course, you know that cakes, cookies, sweets and fizzy drinks aren't ever going to be good for your waistline. But I wonder, are you aware of how much sugary foods and drinks increase your appetite, potentially leading to even more weight gain? Here are three ways that this happens:

1) Sugary foods and drinks provide "empty calories", which don't fill you up

The term empty calories applies to foods and drinks that are high in calories but low in nutrients like vitamins, minerals, fibre, protein or healthy fats. These foods are really easy to eat or drink, and are frequently over-consumed.

It's interesting how much food delivers 195 kcalories, which is 10% of the recommended calorie intake for women or 8% for men:

- 1 small chocolate cookie
- 460ml cola drink
- 590g strawberries

The cookie or cola will do nothing to curb your appetite and will probably increase it, and who can stop at just one cookie? In contrast, not many of us can munch through nearly 600g of strawberries in one go.

Cookies and cola contain only free sugars, which instantly affect blood sugar levels. Interestingly, fruit juice is no better and a glass of fruit juice contains nearly as much free sugar as a cola. When whole fruits are eaten, the sugar is released more slowly as it needs to be digested first and the fibre slows down the transit time. It also takes longer to eat whole fruit compared to just drinking the juice and this gives your brain time to register when you are full.

2) High blood glucose is turned into fat, then stored around your middle

Sugary foods and drinks, such as the cookie and cola mentioned above, will dramatically spike your blood sugar levels, leading to a surge of insulin in an attempt to regulate the sugar rush.

Where does that sugar go?

Normally, it is shuttled by insulin into cells in muscles or organs to provide energy. But with a big sugar rush, insulin has to move it quickly away from the bloodstream and takes it to the liver. There, the excess sugar is converted into fat and stored around your middle; that is where your muffin top, beer belly or love handles come from. (Beer doesn't contain added sugar, but is very high in refined carbohydrates which quickly break down into glucose.)

The big issue is that the fat becomes stored in and around the organs – the liver, pancreas and even the heart – producing a number of factors which increase the risk of heart disease such as inflammation, raised blood pressure and damage to blood vessels.

Another effect of storing the sugary calories that you eat as fat, is that you'll feel hungry, especially if your blood sugar levels fall in response to high insulin levels. Once hormones signal your need to eat, it is very hard to fight against this with willpower.

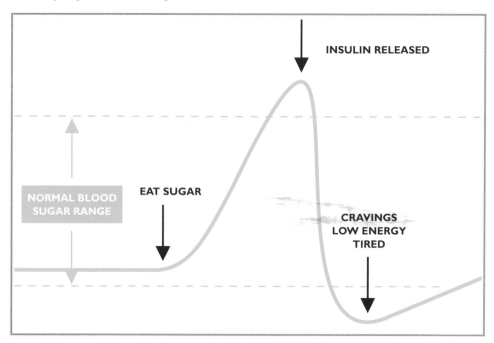

Blood sugar highs and lows with the spike that eating sugar creates

3) High insulin levels affect leptin, the hormone which helps to control appetite

Leptin is produced by your fat cells when you eat, providing feedback to the brain which suppresses your appetite. This is a natural mechanism to prevent overeating. However, when insulin levels are consistently high, the cells also become resistant to the messages from leptin and appetite continues unabated. In response, you keep eating because your hunger doesn't feel satisfied. In summary, when you eat sugary foods regularly, you feel constantly hungry, yet your energy levels are low because the calories you eat are effectively stored as body fat rather than being used for your metabolism.

If you are reading this and feeling that you can get away with eating lots of sugary foods because you are not overweight, then think again. One in seven of people with normal weight have increased internal body fat – this is often described as "thin on the outside, fat on the inside" (TOFI) which also brings with it an increased risk of health complications including type 2 diabetes and cardiovascular problems. The only sure way to protect yourself is to cut the sugary stuff right down.

Are you a TOFI?

The World Health Organisation identified five markers for metabolic health, to help identify whether you are at risk, even if you are not overweight. These are the markers of health:

- Waist measurement less than 35.5 inches for men and 31.5 inches for women
- Blood pressure less than 140/90
- Fasting blood glucose below 5.6 mmol/L
- Fasting triglycerides less than 1.7mmol/L
- Fasting HDL greater than 1.03mmol/L (men) and 1.29mmol/L (women)

In the UK, the NHS offers free health checks to the general public from the age of 40, every 5 years, until the age of 74. These health reviews check not only for diabetes, but also signs of strokes, kidney disease, heart disease and dementia.

Sugar and mental health

Around one in four people in the UK will experience a mental health problem at some time in their life, which could be depression, anxiety, phobias or trauma in addition to other psychiatric disorders. Whilst overall rates are not increasing, there is evidence that some people are finding it harder to cope.

Although mental health is complex and may have many contributing factors, it is interesting to reflect on how sugar can affect how we feel.

We mentioned dopamine earlier, the reward and pleasure hormone that is released when we consume sugary products. In fact, this is similar to how mood altering drugs work, especially when sugar bingeing is regular or even a daily experience. It makes us seek out sweet foods because they make us feel good in the short term. This has been observed in studies where they are seen to stimulate areas of the brain associated with reward and craving. It's not surprising that sugar cravings can be so strong.

What evidence supports a link between sugar and mental health?

Here are a few examples:

• Depression
University College London carried out research in 2017 that found those consuming the highest intake of added sugars had a significantly increased rate of depression, whilst those eating higher quality carbohydrates (less sugar, more fibre, whole grains) had a 30% lower relative risk.

• Mood swings
Profound changes in mood were observed in young healthy individuals associated with the blood sugar dip which follows a sugar binge. Rather than a sugar rush it is more of a sugar crash! We know now that within 30 minutes of having carbohydrates we become more fatigued and within 60 minutes our level of alertness drops (Mantantzis et al 2019).

• Anxiety
Dietary changes involving removing sugar and processed foods resulted in a substantial decrease in anxiety symptoms in just four weeks (Aucoin and Bhardwaj 2016).

Generally, people feel considerably better in their mood and energy levels when they reduce their intake of sugary foods. Whilst this is only part of the mental health conundrum, you are likely to begin to feel more upbeat when you improve your diet.

In this book, we have put the focus on encouraging you to eat nutrient-dense foods that help you to feel fuller for longer. This should make it easier to manage your weight because you'll have more control over your appetite. The foods in the recipes won't dramatically spike your blood glucose levels, which means your insulin and leptin levels can work properly. All in all, this challenge should help you to feel your best.

FALSE BELIEFS

• BRUSH STRAIGHT AFTER EATING AND YOU CAN'T GET TOOTH DECAY
Brushing your teeth immediately after eating does not mean that you can eat what you want. It will not be enough to ensure you do not get tooth decay.

• SUGAR GIVES YOU ENERGY
Sugar *does not* provide you with energy.

• COUNTING CALORIES IS THE KEY TO LOSING WEIGHT
Since the introduction of calorie counting as a method of weight loss, we have continued to see an increase in obesity, type 2 diabetes and other metabolic disorders. Food manufacturers love that we are a calorie-obsessed society because they can write 'only 99 calories' on something like a sugar-sweetened yoghurt and make us believe it is healthy. Remember, when the fat is removed from a product, sugar is usually put in its place. Research has failed to show the benefits of calorie counting. Counting calories can mean you end up thinking about food all the time, which is not good. And not all calories are created equal: your body will recognize and treat them differently. Your body doesn't just digest calories — it digests the minerals, proteins, fats and vitamins that go along with the calories.

1. Start reducing the frequency at which you eat/drink sugar first. This is the best way to reduce your overall sugar intake.

2. Base your meals around vegetables and meat or fish.

3. Stop eating refined grains. We have learnt that whole grains are much better for you, but their slightly more bitter taste and rougher texture are an acquired taste, so if you are used to refined grains, I would suggest mixing whole grains into your refined grains to start with, and then slowly changing the ratios until you are eventually 100% whole grain.

4. Speak to your dentist about how you can modify you and your family's diet to reduce tooth decay. They are trained to give diet advice and help you change habits as part of their care. Plus, they see you regularly and so can help you with your journey.

5. Use a fluoride toothpaste as soon as your children's teeth start to erupt, it is the number one way to reduce dental decay secondary to diet modification.

6. If you suffer from mouth (aphthous) ulcers you may want to consider swapping to an SLS (Sodium Lauryl Sulphate) -free toothpaste. It is a foaming agent that makes some people more prone to mouth ulcers.

3

WHERE

SUGAR

HIDES

co-written with Nutritional Therapist, Jenny Phillips

Our aim with this book is to help you transition away from processed and refined foods and to reclaim your taste buds by adopting easy to prepare and delicious "real food" meals and snacks.

Whilst cooking from scratch does not have the instant convenience of supermarket options, changing your eating habits means you will be quickly rewarded by the satisfaction of how you feel. The many positive likely side effects are: increased energy, better sleep and a liberating sense of not feeling hungry or experiencing cravings most of the time. This is all very common feedback from people who have already made the change.

Sugar can be found in foods where you really wouldn't expect it, which can trip up even those with the best of intentions. It is also important to know how artificial sweeteners work, which is often misunderstood. Armed with the knowledge of where sugar hides, you can be truly in control of your own diet and health.

Labelling

When you cook at home you have complete control over your ingredients and whether you have added any sugar. The trouble is, when purchasing processed foods or eating out, you have no idea whether sugar has been included unless you learn to scan the nutrition labels. Most people take between 4–10 seconds to choose food at the supermarket, so clear labels are important. We are believers in the traffic light system that is on some foods.

Each serving (150g) contains

Energy 1046kJ 250kcal	Fat 3.0g LOW	Saturates 1.3g LOW	Sugars 34g HIGH	Salt 0.9g MED
13%	4%	7%	38%	15%

of an adult's reference intake
Typical values (as sold) per 100g: 697kJ/167kcal

Firstly, look at the total sugars. This will probably be shown in two columns (see illustration on opposite page), per 100g and per portion size (this does vary so do check). The amount per 100g is the best for categorising foods as high, medium or low sugar:

Guidelines per 100g

LOW is classed as having less than 5g of sugar per 100g
MEDIUM is classed as having between 5–22.5g of sugar per 100g
HIGH is classed as having more than 22.5g of sugar per 100g

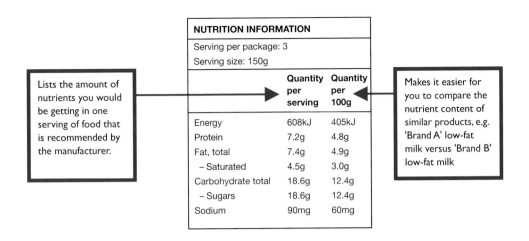

NUTRITION INFORMATION		
Serving per package: 3		
Serving size: 150g		
	Quantity per serving	Quantity per 100g
Energy	608kJ	405kJ
Protein	7.2g	4.8g
Fat, total	7.4g	4.9g
– Saturated	4.5g	3.0g
Carbohydrate total	18.6g	12.4g
– Sugars	18.6g	12.4g
Sodium	90mg	60mg

Lists the amount of nutrients you would be getting in one serving of food that is recommended by the manufacturer.

Makes it easier for you to compare the nutrient content of similar products, e.g. 'Brand A' low-fat milk versus 'Brand B' low-fat milk

The amount of sugar in some of these popular foods may surprise you:

HIGH SUGAR FOODS

Caramel syrup (added to coffee)	79g/100g
Hot chocolate	52g/100g
Cereal bar	28g/100g
Tomato ketchup	23g/100g
Instant porridge with golden syrup	29g/100g
Vanilla ice cream	23g/100g

MEDIUM SUGAR FOODS

Granola	19g/100g
Diet yoghurt	6g/100g
Peanut butter	7g/100g
Apple juice	9g/100g
Korma sauce	7g/100g

Remember that a teaspoon of sugar is about 4g, so would you, for example, put over 10 teaspoons of sugar in your hot chocolate if you had the choice?!

Secondly, study the ingredients list on your packet of food/drink. In the UK, the ingredients listing is ranked by volume, with the largest ingredient first. Scan through for sugar and also its many cousins – yes, sugar comes in many forms. Professor Lustig has written a shopper's guide called "Sugar Has 56 Names" to help people identify the different sources. He also explains that 51% of sugar in our diet is in the foods we expect it to be in and 49% is in foods we don't such as dressings, sauces and bread.

In the UK, the most common names for sugar are:

Sugar including corn sugar and invert sugar
Ingredients ending in 'ose' dextrose, fructose, glucose, high fructose glucose syrup (HFCS), isoglucose, levulose and maltose
Syrups maple, agave, golden
Other honey, molasses

Beware, when several different types of sugar are used in an item of food/drink, they are all given a separate line on the listing. Manufacturers use this as a way of hiding the total amount of added sugars. Another useful way of assessing how much sugar is in a grocery item is to download the Change4Life food scanner app onto your phone. Simply scan a barcode in the grocery store and see how many sugar cubes you will be eating.

Be aware that fruit is quite sugary naturally, hence we limit you to two pieces per day in the upcoming challenge. Berries are generally the least sugary fruits, whereas banana and mango top the sugar charts:

LOW AND HIGH SUGAR FRUITS

(per 100g)	Total Carbs	Sugar	Fibre
Raspberry	12	4	7
Strawberry	8	5	2
Cherry	12	8	2
Kiwi	15	9	3
Orange	12	9	2
Pear	15	9	4
Apple	14	10	2
Blueberries	14	10	2
Pineapple	13	10	1
Banana	23	12	3
Mango	15	14	2

Sugar smart – know where the dangers lie

Despite the huge amount of coverage in the media talking about the dangers of too much sugar, the UK population still massively exceeds the recommended guidelines on page 42 (the guidelines many dental professionals consider too lenient…). Adults are consuming about double (equivalent to 14 teaspoons per day) but children of 4–18 years old are eating or drinking nearly three times the advised amounts.

According to the UK National Diet and Nutrition Survey, the following popular foods and drinks have the highest amount of sugar.

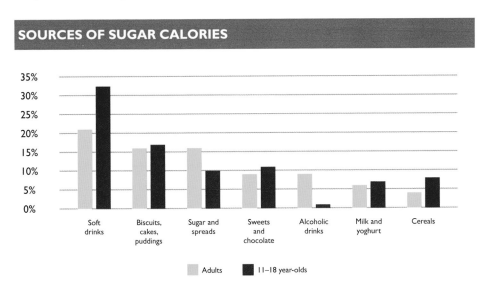

The National Diet and Nutrition Survey (NDNS) from Years 7–8 of the Rolling Programme (2014/15–2015/16)

Soft drinks and sodas

This is the single largest product that drives sugar consumption, accounting for a third of all sugar calories consumed by our children, and one fifth of adult sugar calories. They are so easy to drink and do nothing to satiate you. In fact, as we've discussed (see pages 34–38), they increase hunger by messing up your insulin and blood sugar levels.

Although some drinks like lemonade have less sugar, they often include added artificial sweeteners, which we are also trying to avoid (more on this later).

Don't be deceived by products that are promoted as "natural" such as fruit juice. You still need to check the nutrition label. Fruit juices and smoothies can contain almost as much sugar as cola:

Sugar per 250ml serving:

Fruit smoothie	30g
Cola	26.5g
Apple juice	23g
Lemonade	10.5g

Biscuits, cakes and puddings

If you have a sweet tooth, then doughnuts, custard creams or sticky toffee pudding may be your thing. The occasional indulgence should not be an issue. However, if these things are regulars in your diet, then you are making a sugary rod for your own back because you are likely to be enslaved by sugar cravings which can be hard to resist.

The Rewards Project 2019 survey found that some schools provide dessert every day of the week as part of their lunch offerings. We do not think this is a healthy model for our children, and instead we would recommend that schools limit dessert to one serving per week. School is a place to set up healthy habits for life. There is little point offering healthy eating lessons if you then contradict it with what is actually served at lunchtime.

Sugar, preserves and spreads

Use of sugar in the home, typically added to hot drinks or used within recipes, is an obvious source of the sweet stuff, so cut down where you can.

Recently, there has been a growth in the use of more natural sugars such as organic honey, coconut sugar or maple syrup. The body regards all sugars equally and so overeating any of these will cause the same sugar rush as with white sugar. However, more natural sugars like these do have a better nutritional profile and so are fine to eat occasionally (though we have not included them in the challenge here because we are working on weaning you off your taste for the sweet stuff).

Bear in mind that jams, marmalade, chutneys and pickles can have very high sugar levels – up to 50g per 100g or more. Hazelnut chocolate spread can have as much added sugar as strawberry jam. For a simple first step, try swapping brands as the added sugar levels vary dramatically.

Sweets and chocolate

Sweets and chocolate are often an impulse purchase made when you are looking for a little pick-me-up. Think of the petrol station and the supermarket till where it is almost impossible to pay without having to walk past all of them. They deliver you with a rush of sugar followed by an energy slump around 30 minutes later.

It is a good idea to plan regular meals and/or have a healthy snack handy so that you are less likely to be caught out by the confectionery when you are out and about.

If you like chocolate, then try weaning yourself on to dark chocolate. As the cocoa content increases, the sugar will decrease, leading to a slightly more bitter but rich chocolatey taste. Please try our chocolate taste experiment later in the book (see page 65).

Sugar per 100g:

Milk chocolate	56g
70% dark chocolate	29g
85% dark chocolate	14g

We have written a blog which lists the chocolate with the lowest added sugar:
www.bowlanedental.com/is-chocolate-good-for-you

Alcoholic drinks

Alcohol is the only consumable product in the supermarket that doesn't have a nutrition label, and so it is really difficult to know which drinks contain added sugar. Generally, beers, ciders and liqueurs are sugarier, so settle instead for an occasional glass of dry white or red wine or Champagne! Spirits are low in sugar but the challenge is then finding something low in sugar to drink them with. Again, in this challenge we encourage you to go alcohol free because it will help you reset your taste buds quicker.

Milk and yoghurts

Flavoured yoghurts, especially the low-fat versions, often have added sugars. Instead choose full-fat natural yoghurt and add your own fruit. Raspberries are a good low sugar choice and are available fresh or frozen all year round. Full-fat Greek yoghurt is a good choice as it has a luxurious, rich creaminess that can make you feel full. A small amount of fat from the yoghurt slows the absorption of the fruit sugars so the blood sugar spike is less than with the fruit on its own.

Flavoured milks and commercial ice cream are very high in sugar. As an alternative treat, why not occasionally make your own low-sugar desserts like the ones in the 14-day plan. We have a delicious peanut butter and banana ice cream in our recipes. The banana helps give it a creamy ice cream texture.

Cereals

Kids' breakfast cereals often promote their sweet delights, like frosting and chocolate, in attractive packaging which is very appealing to children. Try and avoid having these in the house to start with if you can. One way of weaning children off these is to mix the no added sugar variety with the normal one. Start at a 25:75 ratio and, over a few weeks, slowly alter the mix until you are completely over to the no added sugar variety. Dried fruits are frequently added to adult cereal products, such as granola, which makes them considerably sugarier. Also, beware of more processed products such as instant porridge, which may contain added sugars in the form of honey or golden syrup. We want you to eventually switch to the alternative breakfast choices we have in this recipe book.

If you are overweight or have diabetes, then you should be aware that cereals contain starches which quickly break down to sugar (as do rice, pasta and potatoes). Although this is less of a problem for your teeth, these starchy foods could dramatically affect your blood sugar levels and promote weight gain. Do look at our breakfast recipes for easy, nutritious and sugar free options which will keep you fuller for longer and feeling more energetic.

Other foods

Other foods like tomato sauces, ketchup and ready meals may contain significant amounts of sugar, so consider making your own sauces and dressings, starting with the recipes in this book. Even some brands of "ready to eat" fish contain added sugar, as can salad dressings and bread. It is hiding everywhere, so always check the label for added sugars or scan the barcode, using the Change4Life sugar app to see how much added sugar a product contains. It pays to become a sugar detective to reduce the exposure to it for you and your family.

Artificial sweeteners – a worthwhile swap, or not?

The focus on sugar in public health has led food manufacturers to reduce calories through non-calorific sweeteners, keeping the same sweet taste but allegedly negating the harms of too much sugar. Some of this has been in direct response to the sugar tax introduced in the UK in 2018 and is already in place in over 35 countries. The tax was initiated after the 2015 World Health Organisation report which detailed the negative health effects of sugar.

The whole area of artificial sweeteners is quite controversial. To the industry, they are potentially a good way out of the damage that sugar is known to do. As a consumer, it feels like we can potentially "have our cake and eat it too" – be able to enjoy the sweetness that we crave without a downside.

When considered as a straight swap, for example, switching a diet cola for a full sugar version, this would seem to make sense. Overall, you have a net reduction in calories, a saving of 97 calories for each substitution made. Similarly, switching a sweetener for 3 tsp sugar in a cup of tea will save 46 calories.

But this is not quite as good as it seems. The catch is that artificial sweeteners still do not reduce appetite and hence the drivers of overeating are maintained. This makes it harder to lose weight if that is your goal, and the small upside in calories saved can be quickly wiped out if accompanied, or followed, by a binge. This is probably why studies into sweetener consumption show either zero-to-modest reduction in weight and a higher incidence of obesity, hypertension, metabolic syndrome, type 2 diabetes and cardiovascular events.

From a dental health perspective, diet soda is still a problem as the drink itself is corrosive to tooth enamel, irrespective of the fact that it doesn't contain sugar. Many "tooth friendly" products contain acidic flavouring that can erode your teeth. You need to be careful about the exposure time. If you are sucking a sugar-free lollipop for several minutes your teeth are again bathed in acid!

Also, your sweet receptors are still overstimulated by artificial sweeteners and so normal foods will taste bitter e.g. broccoli. Consuming artificial sweeteners still alters your palate over time to increase the desire for more sweet foods. We want you to be able to access your full palate, not just the sweet range, and completing this challenge will help you do that.

Can you go cold turkey?

Our preference is for you to forgo the sweet taste, including artificial sweeteners, completely. Hence, the goal is to be able to drink your tea without sugar OR sweeteners; this not only saves the calories but also saves the impact of a sweet taste to drive further cravings. And how about replacing some of your tea/coffee consumption with water? Drinking plenty of water is so important for optimal health, it has zero calories and, what's more, it is completely free if you are drinking in the home or taking a refillable bottle with you.

Going sweet taste free will be the quickest and most efficient way of slaying your sugar urges, stabilising your blood glucose levels and maintaining your energy levels throughout the day. However, if that is too much of an ask, then switching to an artificial sweetener first is at least a step in the right direction. You can then slowly reduce the amount of sweetener until you do not use it at all.

If you enjoy the occasional alcoholic drink, then low-calorie or slimline mixers with sweeteners are a better choice than those with added sugar on balance. Alternatively, add a slice of lemon or lime to fizzy water as a mixer, just remembering that this will be acidic for your teeth. (Side note: Fruit juices are also very acidic and will damage your teeth. Think about having the drink with a meal or neutralising the acid after finishing the drink. You can neutralise this acid with a swill of water, sugar-free chewing gum or a neutral food. It is not advised to brush your teeth immediately after any acidic drink as this will increase the acid damage. If you need to brush straight after, first rinse with some water for 30 seconds and then brush your teeth.)

How we eat is part of the problem

As a generation, we are used to the concept of fast food. We too often think of food just as a way of quickly refuelling, grabbing whatever is easiest and to hand. Planning a meal in advance and sitting down at the table to eat with the rest of the family is not such common practice anymore.

If we feel the start of hunger, we grab a snack or a ready meal and get on with our day, thereby continuing to ride the sugar roller-coaster. We work late at our desks and eat chocolate bars or drink sugar-laden caffeine drinks when the urge strikes. But our bodies like routine, eating at the same times of the day, going to bed and waking up at the same time. Any changes lead to extra stress on the body, which is what we are trying to avoid with this meal plan.

Taking the time to plan a meal that has a good balance of protein, fat and carbohydrate, will make you feel full so there will be no need to snack. My favourite snack used to be cereal bars, I thought they were healthy and would not make me feel hungry again. I didn't realise that most of them were made up of over a third sugar and the ones that didn't were full of artificial sweeteners. This led my body to continue to crave that sweet taste. Since changing my diet, eating more balanced meals and lots more vegetables (you can never eat too many), I have not felt the need to snack.

The three balanced meals per day in the challenge will give your body the routine and balanced diet it really needs. Listen to it over the 14 days and note how your cravings change.

FALSE BELIEFS

YOUR BODY NEEDS SNACKS TO SURVIVE
You do not need to eat between meals. Three well balanced meals each day will provide all of the energy you need and should be enough to keep hunger at bay.

TOP TIPS

1. If you really have to, then switch to artificial sweeteners instead of regular sugar first. Then slowly dial down the sweetness over time so that you are less dependent on it.
2. Really try to wean yourself off sodas and fruit juices as these damage tooth enamel as well as giving your sweet receptors a hit.

4

REWARDING YOURSELF IN A HEALTHY WAY

We have talked about the chemical transmitters in the brain that give us our feelings of pleasure when we eat sugar, but what about how we associate food with pleasure before we eat it, and how can we start to change those associations?

The Collins Dictionary defines a reward as something that you are given, for example, because you have behaved well, worked hard or provided a service to the community.

We are talking about the way the mind reacts to the thought of a stimulus, rather than the stimulus itself. To some people, reading a good book is a reward; for others it is a piece of cake. So, when did we humans start to make the association between sugar and good behaviour or performance? And how does sugar still feature as a reward, especially when we know it is detrimental to our health?

Prehistoric man had more simple rewards than we have today. In ancient Greece, the Olympic games was the first public reward system; the ultimate prize was to win the laurel leaf crown. If you got this you would become a hero in the eyes of the people. We still have Olympic medals today, but humans have developed a far more complex system of rewards and recognition, ranging from Starbucks rewards points to sweets.

In his 1943 paper "The Theory of Human Motivation", American psychologist Maslow explained how humans must have basic physiological needs (such as food, shelter and water) met before being motivated to operate at higher levels. So, think about it, how do you usually reward yourself and your children? Listen to your inner monologue and language before the 14-day challenge. During a boring chore, such as doing the washing up, would you normally tell yourself that "after this, I deserve a biscuit"? How would it be if you chose a different reward like calling a friend on the phone or reading a good book? Later in this chapter, I will list alternative rewards that may give you some inspiration during your 14-day challenge.

Sugar rewards don't just come from you yourself; they are offered to us almost everywhere we go. I am constantly surprised at all these gyms and exercise clubs that offer "protein shakes" after the workout. You push your body at a Barry Bootcamp for an hour and then have a shake packed full of sugar to give you another high after the endorphin rush. All that good cardiovascular work only to be ruined by the sugar. It's probably better for your body overall to avoid the class if you are going to have a shake afterwards! Note that it is especially important to fuel yourself properly after a workout and experts suggest a mixture of healthy carbs and protein within 45 minutes.

The pre-programmed association

Most people replicate the type of rewards they were offered as a child in adulthood. Finish your greens otherwise no dessert, turns into no cake unless chores finished. How were you "pre-programmed" at school or at home? If you did well in a test did you get a chocolate bar? After a relationship break-up, do you now reach for the ice cream tub?

With the rising rates of obesity, diabetes and tooth decay, isn't it time to try and break this pattern? At Rewards Project, we believe the place to start the change is at schools and nurseries. If we can get the healthy eating message across and break the cycle of food and sugar being used early on in life, we will set children on the path to adulthood having a healthier relationship with sugar. For these reasons, we believe schools and nurseries should be sugar-free zones.

We carried out a survey of over 487 schools in the UK and found 10% still reward the children with food/sweets, whilst 48% of schools still celebrate children's birthdays at school with cake and sweets, even though we know they will have it at home as well.

Rewards Project
UK SCHOOL & NURSERY SURVEY 2019

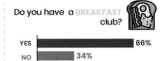

Do you have a BREAKFAST **club?**

YES — **66%**
NO — **34%**

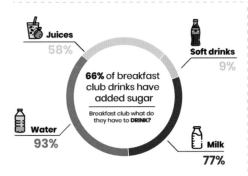

Juices 58%

Soft drinks 9%

66% of breakfast club drinks have added sugar

Breakfast club what do they have to DRINK?

Water 93%

Milk 77%

20% of schools have cereals with high sugar content

CEREALS what is on offer?

Corn Flakes or Rice Crispies	90%
Weetabix	61%
Porridge	35%
Special K or Bran Flakes	12%
Chocolate Shreddies, Cookie Crisp, Sugar puffs or Weetos	11%
Frosties or Crunchy Nut	9%

94% of schools offer desserts with added sugar

Fruit	Cakes/Puddings	Ice cream	Other	Cheese
99%	93%	56%	24%	5%

98% of schools and nurseries provide lunch

Schools on average offer cakes/pudding and sweets for desert on four days per week

Average 4

After sports matches one third of schools provide sugary snacks

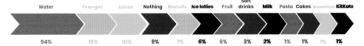

Water	Oranges	Juices	Nothing	Biscuits	Ice lollies	Fruit	Soft drinks	Milk	Pasta	Cakes	Breadsticks	KitKats
94%	18%	10%	9%	7%	6%	6%	3%	2%	1%	1%	1%	1%

After sports matches/days what do you provide?

Schools on average organise cake sales twice a term.

48% of schools allow children to bring in cake and sweets to celebrate birthdays

Bring in cake to school	Bring in sweets for class	Sing Happy Birthday	Get a birthday card	Buy a book for class or library
29%	19%	16%	6%	3%

What happens when it is a child's birthday?

BUY For schools with a tuck shop, 84% sell snacks with added sugar

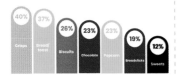

Crisps	Bread/toast	Biscuits	Chocolate	Popcorn	Breadsticks	Sweets
40%	37%	26%	23%	23%	19%	12%

When children do well in test or complete a good piece of work **10%** of schools reward them with food or sugar.

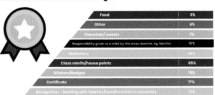

Food	3%
Other	6%
Chocolate/sweets	7%
Responsibility given to a child by the class teacher, eg. Monitor	19%
Stationery	24%
Class merits/house points	65%
Stickers/Badges	75%
Certificate	77%
Recognition – Meeting with teacher/head/mention in assembly	77%

When they do well in tests or complete a good piece of work, what do they receive?

Survey data from **487 schools**

You can read our full report at:
www.rewardsproject.org/report

Non-food rewards

There are many alternative rewards that you and your family could transition to. I have divided these up into experiences and time. If you think back over your highlights of the previous month, I doubt the best of those was when you ate that extra portion of dessert. Most of our fondest memories are related to experiences, especially of ones that are shared with others.

Experiences

A walk outside
Fresh flowers
Dance class
Taking a bath
Spa day
A massage
Reading a book or magazine
Listening to music or a podcast
Going on a bike ride
Screen time
Theatre
Cinema tickets (One of the best rewards we gave at our Bow Lane practice was a pair of cinema tickets to all the team members. It doesn't matter what salary you are on; this was a treat for everyone.)

Time

With friends and family
With your children – not looking at your phone!
Shopping
Meditation
Cup of tea/coffee
Relaxing in the garden or on the sofa

With children, depending on their ages, simple things like certificates, stickers, stationery, a book, bookmark, small toys, craft kits, jewellery and balls are great fun. As are games like den-making, digging in the garden and hide and seek. Rewards do not always need to cost anything. You could speak to your family and discuss how they would like to be rewarded.

Rewards versus recognition

Let us look at how we are rewarded at work, as we spend a third of our adulthood here. Do you have a sweet drawer that you rummage in when you finish a difficult task or are bored and no one is watching? In Chapter 6, we are going to show you how to break those habits. At work, how does your manager encourage you? At Bow Lane Dental, we have things like employee of the quarter awards, appraisal meetings and salary increases – but is that enough? Most people want a simple thank you.

Rewards and recognition are both important but very different. Rewards are more appropriate for managing behaviours or meeting standards, such as good timekeeping or cleaning your room. We also need to be careful when removing rewards because they often turn into expectations or even entitlements. Recognition is when someone goes above and beyond, uses their initiative or creativity. These are usually intrinsically driven and whether they are recognized or not, they will continue. Research shows that the most important aspect of recognition is that it is done timely, sincerely and ideally in view of our teammates.

In the context of this challenge – think about how you are rewarding yourself or colleagues. Is it always with food or sugar? Could you all go out bowling when you hit a target rather than bringing in a box of doughnuts? One of the best ways to design a rewards programme at work is to sit down with your team and find out what motivates them.

Think about it honestly. Have you promised yourself a reward for completing this challenge? Can you offer your family members recognition for completing it successfully?

FALSE BELIEFS

SUGAR IS A WAY OF REWARDING THE BODY
Sugar does nothing to reward or look after your body. Find other ways to reward yourself.

TOP TIPS

• Think about how you currently reward yourself.
• How about getting a group of parents together to reduce sugar at your kids' school? The Rewards Project has lots of free resources to help you.
• You can never say too many sincere "thank yous" to others.
• Before you design a reward programme, work out the behaviours you want to encourage and the outcome you desire.

5

DISCOVER YOUR FULL

RANGE

OF TASTE

What is taste?

Taste helps us to determine whether food is nutritious and safe to eat. It has a protective function to avoid potentially toxic (bitter), indigestible substances and food that has gone off. It is a combination of the smell, texture, appearance and temperature of food/drink and how these all combine to signal to your brain.

Various different things can affect your sense of taste. Have you noticed that when you have a cold or blocked nose food tastes different? The largest number of taste buds can be found on your tongue and palate, but we even have taste receptors in our guts! We used to think different parts of the mouth had different receptors, but we now realise this was wrong. Our taste changes as we age and as we grow older it grows more complex. Babies are born with the ability to detect sweet but cannot detect salt until about four months old. There is definitely a genetic inclination to like sweetness (Keskitalo et al 2007), but the degree of liking for sweetness and the cravings varies from person to person.

The consensus is that we have five taste receptors:

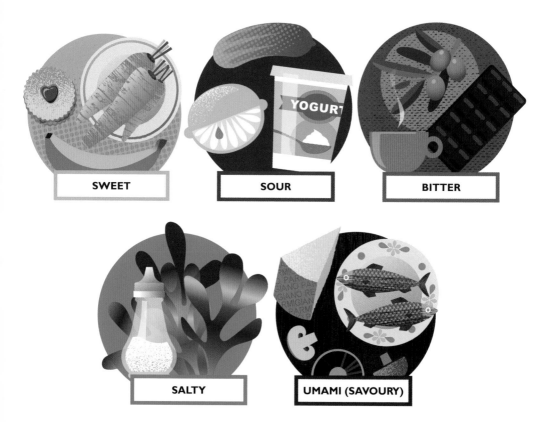

SWEET

SOUR

BITTER

SALTY

UMAMI (SAVOURY)

We also know fat gives texture to food and, more recently, it has been thought that we might actually have a sixth taste receptor for fat.

How to make food tasty without sugar

Here comes the important bit: A study from Bartolotto (2015) has shown that just six days of consuming less added sugar will change your taste, allowing your palate to appreciate a whole range of flavours rather than just sweet.

Making changes to your eating habits can feel a bit scary. One concern may be whether you will still enjoy food. We are actually all programmed to seek variety in order to obtain all the nutrients our bodies require, so use this challenge to try some new foods. Here are some tips to help:

1. Enjoy good quality fats

Unfortunately, fat has been maligned since the 1950s, especially after the dietary guidelines were introduced in 1980. But many experts now believe that the war against fat, and the consequent rise in sales of refined carbohydrates or sugar to substitute calories, has been a disaster. The evidence for this conclusion is in the massive growth in diet-related diseases.

Increasing your fat intake helps to make foods delicious and satiating, making you feel fuller, which helps to reduce cravings. Because of this, fats can actually help to manage your weight as well as helping to build a healthy brain and nervous system, make hormones and provide fat-soluble vitamins. We encourage you to replace vegetable oils, that provide no flavour, with delicious oils such as olive oils and butter. Later on, we will discuss the oils and fats you should stock in your kitchen (see page 74).

The importance of fat-soluble vitamins is also massively underestimated by the low-fat brigade. Healthy bones and teeth need vitamins A, D and K2. Animal products are a great source of these vitamins, especially full-fat dairy products like cheese and yoghurt. Vitamin E is another fat-soluble vitamin that is a powerful antioxidant, protecting your cells from damage. It is found in nuts, seeds and oily fish.

2. Add good quality salt (such as rock salt or sea salt)

Here we are busting another dietary myth: that salt is bad for us. The original research showed that high sodium together with low potassium intake was bad for blood pressure and hence a cardiovascular risk. It is the ratio of sodium to potassium that is important – but the message got simplified. Yes, if you are eating a poor quality ultra-processed diet with low or no vegetables (low potassium), you cannot afford to add salt. But, if you follow this plan, then your food will be high in potassium, which is abundant in natural foods, especially vegetables, and you can absolutely afford to enhance the flavour with salt. If you want to read more about the science of salt, I highly recommend *The Salt Fix* by Dr James DiNicolantonio.

3. Go large on herbs and spices

These are nature's flavour enhancers and pharmacy rolled up into one. Take cinnamon, which helps to improve insulin sensitivity and hence blood sugar regulation and vanilla, it gives a natural distinctive sweetness and can have a therapeutic, calming effect. Herbs are little powerhouses when it comes to providing flavour, vitamins and minerals, so do include them whenever you can. They can be easily grown in your kitchen or garden to ensure you have a ready supply.

4. Use different cooking methods

In 1912, the chemist Louis-Camille Maillard found that foods containing protein had a molecular change at around 140°C, which affected their taste. This helps explain how foods brown and take on different flavours as they cook. Think of seared steak, crisp fish skin and toasted nuts. Cooking has an effect on the nutrients in foods, with some increasing and others not. For optimal health it is important to have a variety of fresh and cooked vegetables. Vegetables like carrots release more nutrients when cooked, whereas red peppers are better raw. Read on for more information on this.

Ways to cook vegetables

We encourage you to eat a multitude of veggies in this book – there are so many wonderful varieties to try and so much you can do with them to make them delicious. Different vegetables benefit from different cooking methods, so I've broken this down for you here. Note that steaming and blanching tend to retain more nutrients than other cooking methods.

Stir-frying

This is the fastest way to cook vegetables, ensuring they keep their texture and taste. The secret is to get the wok or frying pan to a very high temperature. The vegetables in a stir-fry need to be thinly sliced and evenly sized so that the outsides do not burn before the insides cook. Start with the vegetables that need the longest cooking (due to density and moisture content) and keep them moving so they do not burn. Do not overfill your stir-fry pan, otherwise the contents will steam rather than fry; cook in batches instead if you need to.

Ideal for: mushrooms, carrots, sugar snap peas, courgettes, broccoli, onions, peppers and baby corn.

Sautéing

This is similar to stir-frying but is done over a medium-high heat and for slightly longer until the vegetables are softened and have a bit of colour. A little oil is needed to lubricate the pan and the vegetables should be tossed from time to time. Again, the vegetables should be cut into equal sized pieces and do not crowd the pan.

Ideal for: asparagus, mushrooms, peppers, courgettes, onions and green beans.

Boiling

Boiling is a quick cooking method, especially for root vegetables, and is easy to control. Use as little water as possible and avoid overcooking, which can kill all the nutrients and flavour. Adding salt to the water when boiling vegetables actually makes vegetables cook faster as it helps break down their cell walls, making them more tender. Usually, you would add the vegetables to a pan of boiling water, quickly bring back to the boil, cover, then simmer until just tender. With potatoes, parsnips and carrots, start with cold water and boil them gently. A lot of vitamin C is lost through boiling, so it is a good idea to retain the water and use it as a tasty soup base. Both steaming and microwaving actually retain more nutrients than boiling, so make sure you don't boil all your veg!

Ideal for: broccoli, cauliflower, potatoes, carrots and parsnips.

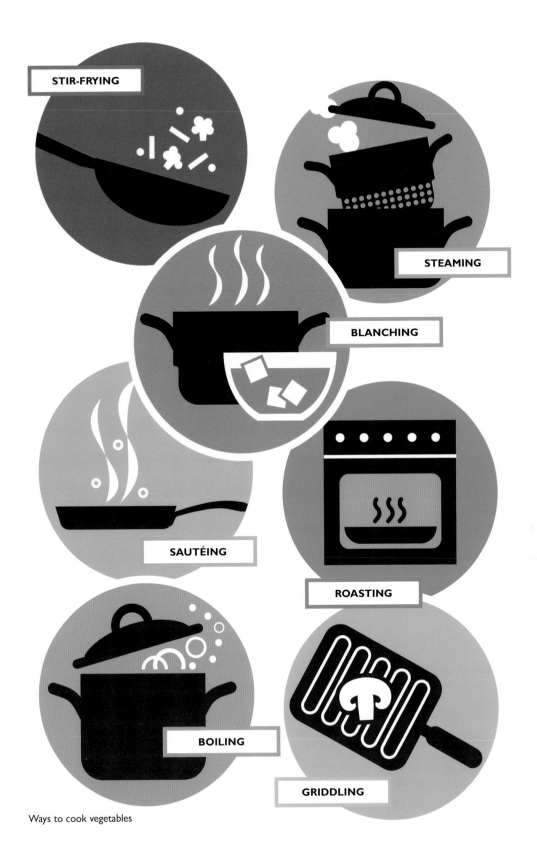

STIR-FRYING

STEAMING

BLANCHING

SAUTÉING

ROASTING

BOILING

GRIDDLING

Ways to cook vegetables

Steaming

Steaming vegetables is a good way of retaining their flavour, colour and nutrients. Because they are not immersed in water, more nutrients, like vitamin C, are retained. You can either buy a tiered steamer pan or use a steamer basket set inside a normal saucepan. Simply boil the water, add the vegetables to the steamer basket and cover with a tight-fitting lid. The food must be loosely packed to allow the steam to circulate. When ready, immediately remove the steam basket and take the lid off to prevent the vegetables from overcooking. You can also steam vegetables in the oven in their own juices. Just wrap in baking paper or tin foil and then cook them in the oven at 180°C until tender.

Ideal for: broccoli, cauliflower, carrots, green beans and asparagus.

Blanching

Blanching is plunging vegetables into boiling water to partially cook them. It is used to help seal in the colour, flavour and nutrients of the vegetables. It also softens vegetables, such as tomatoes, making it easier to peel the skin off. Blanching is also used to remove the bitterness of vegetables before they are frozen, as this destroys the enzymes that cause deterioration and retains more vitamins. Just add vegetables to a pan of boiling water, return to the boil and cook for one minute. The time varies depending on what your purpose is. Then plunge the drained vegetables into iced water to stop the cooking process. Drain and pat dry with kitchen paper before using or freezing.

Ideal for: green beans, fresh peas, mange tout, asparagus, cauliflower.

Roasting

Roasting intensifies flavours and causes natural sugars to caramelise, creating a crisp outer coating and a tender centre. Vegetables should be first tossed in oil or melted butter, seasoned and flavoured with sprigs of fresh hardy herbs (tarragon, rosemary, thyme etc.), then spread in a single layer in a baking tray at roasted at 180–200°C. Root vegetables and squashes need longer in the oven at a higher temperature (about 45 minutes), whereas things like Brussels sprouts and broccoli only need about 25 minutes at a slightly lower temperature. The vegetables should be tossed or turned at least once during cooking.

Ideal for: tomatoes, peppers, asparagus, squash, courgettes and root vegetables.

Griddling

Griddling, like barbecuing, is a direct heat cooking method, which gives a crisp coating and a tender centre. Make sure your griddle pan is really hot before you start. Slice the vegetables to an even size, brush with olive oil and sit them flat in the pan. Avoid pricking them while they are cooking, as this will release their juices and dry them out. To get the chargrilled stripe effect, don't move them, just turn them once.

Ideal for: aubergines, portobello mushrooms, courgettes, peppers and onions.

How to cook grains

Grains are another spectacularly nutritious and delicious type of food and understanding how to cook with them is key to a healthy diet. Always read the packet instructions first, but generally the cooking method is as follows: rinse the grains first until the water no longer changes colour. Put the drained grains in a heavy-based saucepan with a tight-fitting lid. Add the water (see ratios below), bring to the boil and then simmer until the liquid has been absorbed. The exact cooking time depends on the age of the grain, the variety and the pans you cook with. Keep an eye on them and when they are tender and tasty, they are done. To speed up the cooking time, you can pre-soak grains in water for a few hours first. You can also batch cook and then keep in an airtight container in the fridge for 3–4 days.

Similar to cooking rice, the tricky bit is getting the grain to water ratio right.

Those ratios – water first – are:

- **2:1** rice, buckwheat, bulgur, millet, quinoa, rolled oats
- **3:1** pearl barley, farro
- **4:1** wild rice

Eat real food

Throughout this challenge, I want to encourage you to eat real food whenever possible. I mean by this, food that has been cooked from scratch and does not need a label. Look out for locally produced, in season, organic, naturally grown and grass-fed produce. Shop at a local farmers' market or in a farm shop if and when you can. Not only will the food taste better, as it has not travelled thousands of miles, it is better for the environment and you will also get to meet the people who grew it. You see, the flavour and nutrient content of fruit and vegetables dramatically changes depending on how they are grown, harvested and handled.

University of California has shown that plants lose 30% of their nutrients within three days of them being harvested. It is all down to a process called 'respiration', as they continue to live and convert their sugars and oxygen into carbon dioxide and water. So, you want to try and buy produce that is as fresh as possible. If you are not going to eat what you buy within a couple of days, then it is probably better to freeze it, which will lock in the nutrients. Some vegetables are actually better for you bought frozen because they are picked and harvested at their peak. Buying frozen fruit and veg also allows us to buy produce at a cheaper price, save preparation time (think of shelling those peas) and consume out of season produce. Nutrients in frozen vegetables also degrade over time, so we recommend using them within 3 months. Some of the best frozen produce to have on hand is: broccoli, carrots, cauliflower, peas, green beans, spinach, sweetcorn, sweet potatoes and mixed berries.

Some fruits and vegetables are safe to refrigerate, but for others it accelerates their demise and reduces their flavour.

Store at room temperature

Fruits
Apples, bananas, grapefruit, lemons, limes, mandarins, mangoes, melons, oranges, papayas, pineapple, plantain, pomegranates, watermelons.

Vegetables and herbs

Basil (stems in water), cucumbers*, aubergine*, peppers*, garlic, ginger, turnips, onions, potatoes, pumpkins, sweet potatoes, tomatoes, winter squashes.

*can be kept in the fridge for up to 3 days
Note: Potatoes need to be stored in the dark to avoid them turning green.

Store in the fridge

Fruits

Apricots, pears, all berries, cherries, figs, grapes

Vegetables and herbs

Artichokes, asparagus, green beans, beetroots, broccoli, Brussels sprouts, cabbage, carrots, cauliflower, celery, herbs (except basil), leafy greens, leeks, lettuce, mushrooms, peas, radishes, spinach, sprouts, squash, sweetcorn.
Note: Make sure the fridge is not too cold or this will also speed up the demise of the produce.

Mini taste experiments

As mentioned earlier in the book, it takes as little as six days of cutting back on sugar and processed/refined foods to start to regain your taste buds. However, it takes a bit longer to start to form a habit, which is why we chose 14 days for this challenge. Some people believe it takes as much as 30 days to lock a habit into place, but our hope is that once you notice how great your body feels after the 14 days, you will continue – not just for 30 days, but for life.

Here are two interesting mini taste experiments to help you appreciate your taste buds and how your body digests food:

Bread chewing

As discussed earlier in the book, bread is a carbohydrate and breaks down to sugar in the body. For this experiment you can use any bread.

Take a bite-size chunk of bread and put it in your mouth. Close your eyes and chew SLOWLY. Do not swallow it yet. Chew it for 2 minutes and notice the change in taste. It may start off bitter and dry, but it will get increasingly sweet – stay with it! After 2 minutes, you may either swallow it or spit it out.

So, what is happening, why does it taste sweet? It is the enzymes in your saliva (particularly amalyase) breaking down the starch in the bread to produce sugar. This is what happens in your body every time you eat bread, but you do not notice it as you have long since swallowed it and gone on to the next bite!

Chocolate melting

This is my favourite one. Take a small piece (just one square) of chocolate, any type, but it works better with 70% cocoa solids and above. Close your eyes and smell it for ten seconds, then put it on the centre of your tongue and let it melt. Do not chew or swallow, just let it dissolve. Try and make out all the flavours: it might taste fruity, floral, earthy or spicy. Notice how the flavours change as the chocolate

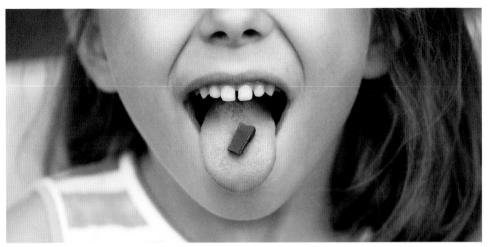

Try melting chocolate on your tongue to fully appreciate its taste

melts. What about the texture of the chocolate? Is it smooth, grainy? Can you taste the fat? With good quality chocolate, the flavour will stay with you for a few minutes after it has melted. Try this with a couple of different types of chocolate and see which you prefer. Hopefully you will appreciate chocolate more and take your time the next time you eat it!

FALSE BELIEFS

• **FROZEN VEGETABLES ARE LESS HEALTHY THAN FRESH ONES**
Freezing vegetables is a way of locking in nutrients, which fresh vegetables can lose day by day.

• **BEING VEGAN OR VEGETARIAN IS ALWAYS MORE HEALTHY**
Not necessarily, it all depends on what food you eat as a vegan/vegetarian. For example, fried or processed veggie burgers and chips are harmful in their own way. Research suggests that one of the main reasons vegans/vegetarians are healthier is that they are more health conscious overall than the general population. Whether you choose to consume animal products or not, the best thing you can do for your body is to consciously make an effort to eat a variety of natural and unprocessed foods to get the vitamins and nutrients you need. You should still be looking at the quality of the foods in your diet. If you follow a vegan diet you may need to take some additional supplementation which you cannot get through a vegan diet, such as B12. Some delicious and healthy vegan and vegetarian recipes are included in this book, look out for those marked **V** (vegan) and V (vegetarian).

TOP TIPS

• Don't wash fruits and vegetables until you're ready to eat them.
• Put kitchen paper between layers of berries to extend storage time.

6

CHALLENGE
PREPARATION

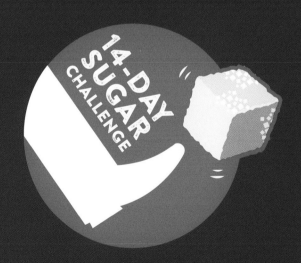

It is nearly time to get started with the challenge, but before you start you need to plan to succeed. A small amount of preparation will give you a greater chance of completing the challenge and breaking your cycle with sugar. You will then start to reap the health benefits and get back control of your life. This is not a diet; it is a way of eating real foods and discovering your full range of taste again. At the end of the 14 days, you are likely to reintroduce certain foods back into your diet, however, hopefully you will have learnt to listen to your body to see what nourishes and energises it and what does not.

At the start of the book, you completed a health scorecard so we know where you started. You will complete the same scorecard at the end of the challenge to see your progress.

With the help of a dietitian and nutritionist, I have complied a simple list of what you can and can't eat during this challenge. Some sugar 'detoxes' are much more restrictive and do not allow any grains or fruits, however, we want this plan to be as accessible as possible and having a less restrictive plan will allow more people to complete this and start to feel the health benefits. Once this challenge is over, you may decide to remove further things from your diet, we encourage you to try this slowly and one food group at a time so you can see what works best for your body.

You will notice a change in taste over the 14 days, some people really notice a difference after just six days, whereas others take longer to experience this shift. The recipes are a guide, so feel free to modify them as your taste changes. For example, we have a delicious recipe for chocolate cake in week one that uses 85% cocoa solids chocolate. Over time, you may find that too sweet and want to increase it to 90% or perhaps 100%. This is your journey to better heath and these kinds of details are up to you.

Sugar withdrawal

During the challenge, you may experience psychological and/or physical withdrawal symptoms from sugar, depending on how much of it you currently eat. For most people, this will start after two or three days. Remember that it is only temporary, and you will feel MUCH better at the end of the challenge. If you mentally prepare yourself for these obstacles by studying the information below, you will find it much easier to cope when the symptoms occur.

Psychological withdrawal

We touched on some of this in Chapter 2 when talking about rewards. When the impulse to reach for something sweet comes up in the next 14 days, try to plan what you can do instead. Some of our poor eating choices occur simply when we are bored. Rather than just rely on your willpower, think about what your immediate responses to a sugar craving could be:

- **Drink a glass of water** – this feeling of low energy could well be your body's way of telling you it is just dehydrated.
- **Find a favourite herbal tea to enjoy** – I love chamomile.
- **Get some fresh air** – even a two-minute walk will energise you.
- **Meditate** – if you have never tried it before there are plenty of apps out there to help you get started, one is Insight Timer.
- **Slowly count to ten** – bide your time and see if the craving passes.

Changing behaviour takes time, so don't be too hard on yourself, especially if you have eaten sugar all your life. It may take a few attempts to get it right. It is important to understand your own personal motivation taking on the challenge: is it a response to a recent health scare? Do you want to avoid getting ill or stop dental disease? Hold these motivations in your mind when a sugar craving comes up and remember why you are doing it in the first place.

Physical withdrawal

Some physical symptoms can occur after two or three days of reduced sugar. It can affect your mood, vision, sleep and some people experience headaches or flu-like symptoms. Others get minor skin irritation or acne. It is only your body removing all the toxins and these will pass and get better. You may be tired and grumpy, so warn your family in advance if they are not doing it with you. Drinking loads of water (eight glasses) a day, plus getting daily fresh air and exercise, really helps this process.

Control your environment

A great first step is to create an environment at home that will support you throughout your challenge. Minimise your access to sugary foods and surround yourself with fresh and tempting healthy produce instead. This will make it so much easier and you will not have to rely on your willpower alone to complete the challenge.

WHAT IS ALLOWED		
MEAT	SEAFOOD	EGGS
DAIRY (FULL-FAT)	VEGETABLES	NUTS AND SEEDS
FRUITS (NO MORE THAN 2 PORTIONS A DAY) *		
WHOLE GRAINS (NO MORE THAN 3 SERVINGS A WEEK) **		
HERBS AND SPICES		COFFEE AND TEA
SPARKLING WATER (UNSWEETENED)		

* See page 44 for a comparison of the sugar content of different fruits
** Such as brown rice, wild rice, barley, buckwheat, bulgur (cracked wheat), millet, oatmeal, popcorn, whole wheat or spelt pasta, bread and flour

WHAT IS NOT ALLOWED		
READY MEALS	PROCESSED FOODS	BREAKFAST CEREALS
ALCOHOL	LOW-FAT DAIRY	SWEETENERS *
CARBONATED DRINKS, FRUIT JUICES, SPORTS OR ENERGY DRINKS		
VEGETABLE OILS (SUCH AS RAPESEED, SUNFLOWER AND PEANUT OILS)		
REFINED GRAINS (SUCH AS WHITE RICE, BREAD AND PASTA) **		
CONDIMENTS (SUCH AS KETCHUP AND MAYONNAISE)		

* Including in toothpaste and in chewing gum!
** Anything made from white flour

The Sweet Sweeper

I devised this simple exercise to enable you to banish sweet things from your immediate surroundings prior to undertaking the challenge.

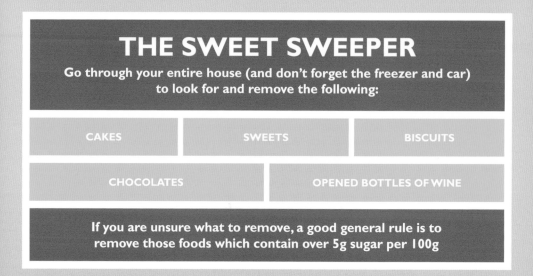

THE SWEET SWEEPER

Go through your entire house (and don't forget the freezer and car) to look for and remove the following:

CAKES	SWEETS	BISCUITS

CHOCOLATES	OPENED BOTTLES OF WINE

If you are unsure what to remove, a good general rule is to remove those foods which contain over 5g sugar per 100g

Pile the foods/drinks up on the table and take a picture of them and upload it to social medias with the tag #SweetSweeper and throw them out! I know you may feel that this is wasteful and, if you prefer to give them to a friend or neighbour or deliver to a homeless charity or food bank that is fine, but just get them out of your house to make room for all the delicious healthy foods.

One item that is often overlooked is sugar-sweetened medicines. Sugar is commonly added to liquid codeine, antibiotics, cough medicines and children's medicines. A lot of manufacturers are slowly bringing out sugar-free versions like Calpol. It is better than the full sugar version, but we are disappointed that they replace the sugar with artificial sweeteners. Next time your doctor prescribes medication, do ask for the sugar-free version. If you are having these, especially on a long-term basis, make sure you take them at mealtimes and at least one hour before bed, as your saliva has more time to clear the sugar from your mouth.

Alcohol

As this challenge also involves no alcohol for the two weeks, perhaps you should think about cutting down in the weeks before you start and decide what drink you will choose instead of your usual alcoholic drink. Do not worry. You will be able to start drinking again after the challenge, but we have found to get the quickest change no alcohol is allowed in these 14 days. Alcohol gives many people the munchies and weakens their resolve. There are many resources to help you cut down, such as Club soda or Soberistas.

Shopping lists and kitchen essentials

All the delicious recipes are in the next two chapters and so it may be worth skipping to the next chapter to check the recipes that most appeal to you and then you can make sure you stock up with all the ingredients to get started. Let us talk about the kitchen essentials; if you do not have any of these items you may also want to add these to your shopping list.

To get full flavours and bring a dish to life without adding sugar you will need to involve herbs and spices. In the previous chapter, I explained how they improve taste of foods and drinks. You can be as liberal as you want with fresh herbs but take more care with dried herbs and only use the directed amount as too much can give an unpleasant taste. Store dried herbs in an airtight container in a cool, dark place.

Also, depending on the herbs, they need to be added at different times in the cooking process as some of the herbs are more delicate and can be easily damaged. Mint, basil, chives, coriander, dill, parsley and tarragon are more delicate and are best added towards the end of cooking or used as a garnish. Bay, oregano, rosemary, sage and thyme can be added at the beginning and cooked in oil or fat to help release more of their flavour.

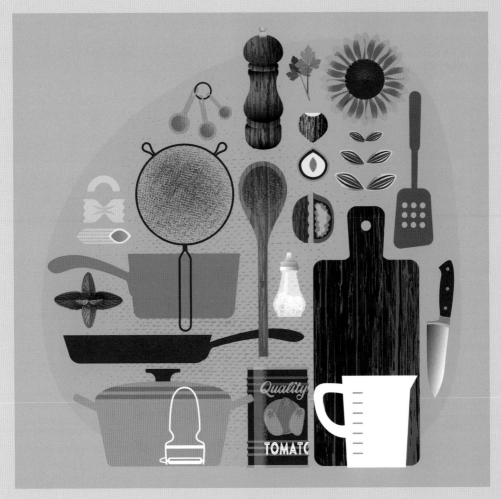

My go-to spices

Salt Not really a spice, but my first port of call when enhancing a dish's flavour and especially when we want to reduce sugar. Not only does it have its own flavour, but it affects how we experience other tastes. You will see later how we use it in the chocolate cake recipe

Pepper Adds heat and depth of flavour

Cinnamon Regulates blood sugar and is anti-inflammatory. Easy way to make foods appear to be "sweeter" without damage to your body

Cumin Usually used in curries and stews

Chilli powder Adds a spicy kick to dishes

Ginger Works well in sweet and savoury dishes, cakes, smoothies, stir-fries and curries

Garlic Antioxidant and, depending on how it is prepared, you can control the level of sweetness it adds to the dish

Lemongrass Used whole in stews, curries and in teas. Chop and use to make marinades and soups or add to stir-fries

Cardamom For both sweet and savoury dishes. Use sparingly as it's strong. It can combat bad breath (chew a pod after meals or drink cardamom tea in the morning)

Garam masala A mixture of spices that aids digestion. We have used it in our vegetable curry

Kaffir lime Used to infuse curries, soups, stir-fries or stock with spiced-citrus flavour. We have used it in our Thai green chicken curry

Turmeric Brings warmth and colour to dishes. It has anti-inflammatory effects. We have used it in our vegetable curry.

Vanilla Not just for ice cream and cakes. We use it in our granola, crumble, rice pudding, peanut butter and banana ice cream recipes

Nutmeg Buy nutmeg whole and grate it as you need it, to get the best flavour. It has various health benefits including its use to treat bad breath and toothache. We have used it in our baked fish and creamed spinach recipe

Cacao powder Do not confuse this with cocoa powder. Also from the cacao plant. Cocoa powder is processed at a higher temperature and often has sugar added, so check the label before you buy. Cacao is a superfood that can help to regulate blood sugar levels. We use it in our chocolate cake, chocolate quinoa and our chilli

My go-to dried herbs

Oregano Used to flavour sauces and marinate meats. We use it in our scramble, meatballs and tomato ketchup

Thyme Many varieties. We use common garden thyme in our brunch and lemon chicken recipes

Basil Added towards end of cooking for flavour

Parsley Used in stock and as a subtle garnish

Mint Helps ease digestive ailments and eases symptoms of irritable bowel syndrome. Garnish in drinks and desserts. A great herbal tea

Rosemary Great with meats

Coriander Wonderful source of vitamins K, A and C in curries and as a garnish

Nuts and seeds

Almonds A good source of fibre and protein, plus contain vitamin E, selenium, zinc, calcium, magnesium and B vitamins

Cashews Lower in fat and with a higher protein and carbohydrate content than most other nuts. Full of healthy monounsaturated fats, great for diabetic patients

Flaxseeds (linseeds) Great for protein and fibre. Ideally grind just before eating to get the full benefit

Pine nuts Like the above nuts, they are high in beneficial monounsaturated fats, magnesium and vitamin E. We use them in our pesto recipe

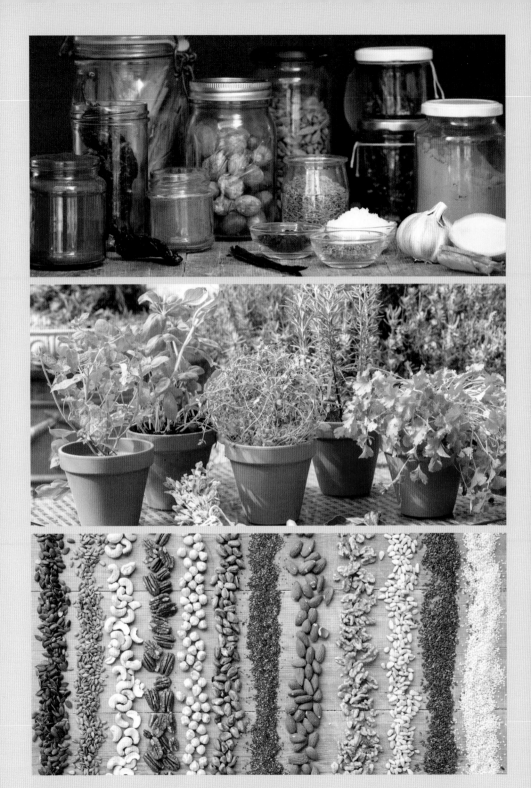

A good range of storecupboard spices will give you the perfect weaponry to enhance dish after dish. Herbs can easily be grown in pots in your garden or on the windowsill. And nuts and seeds will bring flavour and texture.

Pecans High in vitamin E. We have used them in our crumble

Walnuts Full of antioxidants and rich in omega-3 fatty acids. We use them in our Caesar salad and carrot cake

Hazelnuts Hazelnuts are a good source of dietary fibre and help lower cholesterol. We use them in our chocolate quinoa and bircher muesli

Pistachios Full of essential vitamins and minerals, high in protein and an excellent source of healthy fats. They've been shown to improve blood sugar, lower blood pressure and improve markers of cardiovascular health. We use them in our halloumi and spinach salad

Chia seeds High in protein. These are used in our fruit and yoghurt sundae, rice pudding, porridge and our sweet smoothie recipe

Sunflower seeds Rich in vitamin E, magnesium and selenium

Pumpkin seeds Full of zinc. Used in our granola and bircher muesli recipes

Sesame seeds Used in our tuna poke, salmon and bircher muesli recipes. Sesame oil is also a healthier alternative to normal vegetable oil, adding a nutty taste to many of our dishes

Dried goods

Pulses An edible seed that grows in a pod. If you buy tinned pulses, check the label and try to choose ones that have no added sugar. They are great sources of protein, fibre, vitamins and minerals. Ones we have used in our recipes include beans, lentils and chickpeas

Whole grain pasta There are now so many whole grain varieties available

Whole grain rice Unlike white rice, whole grain includes the fibrous bran and the nutritious germ parts of the grain

Porridge oats Vitamin- and mineral-rich and a great slow-release complex carbohydrate

Soba (100% buckwheat) noodles A high-fibre noodle with a lovely nutty taste

Cornflour An invaluable thickening agent for sauces and soups

Wholemeal self-raising flour Gives texture and flavour to cakes and muffins and is a great alternative to white self-raising flour

Oils, vinegars, butters, sauces

Extra virgin olive oil For drizzling and dressings

Coconut oil Can be eaten raw and you can cook with it

Groundnut or avocado oil Ideal for stir-frying

Sesame oil For cooking, but also adds a wonderful nutty aroma and flavour to dishes

Balsamic vinegar For cooking and adding acidic flavour to salads

Apple cider vinegar A really flavoursome vinegar with great health benefits

Rice wine vinegar A vinegar milder and sweeter in taste than most other vinegars

Butter Adds flavour and can be used to fry at low heat. Ideally unsalted so you can then decide how much salt to add to a recipe

Unsweetened nut butters e.g. cashew, almond or peanut High in protein and a great choice to elevate a smoothie or porridge

Soy sauce Strong umami taste for enriching sauces or to be enjoyed neat as a dipping sauce

Dijon mustard A sharp and tangy mustard that works well for dressings

Tin whole plum tomatoes A storecupboard essential for all manner of sauce and stew bases

Tomato purée Thicker than sauce or paste and with a greater depth of tomato flavour

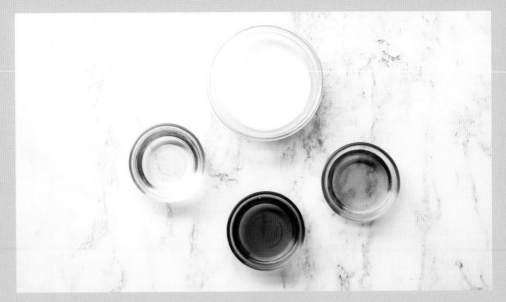

A simple selection of oils

Utensils and equipment

A dozen or so bits of essential kitchen equipment will set you on your way to recreating the recipes in this book and to learning a wonderful variety of healthy new dishes. You won't need to spend lots of money to assemble all that you will need, but having all of this to hand will be one of the best investments for your health you can make.

Blender (can be a hand-held stick blender); Knives (ideally a chef's knife and a paring knife); Chopping board; Mixing bowls; Saucepans (small, medium and large); non-stick frying pan (24cm); Casserole dish; Measuring jug; Scales; Sieve; Measuring spoons; Slotted spoon; Metal spatula; Y-shaped peeler; Metal tongs; Pestle and mortar; Wooden spoons; Balloon whisk; Grater; Greaseproof paper/baking paper; Tin foil

Cooking skills

Depending on your level of cooking ability to start with, you may have more or less to learn in this challenge. One of the best things you can do for your health is learn to cook – if you cannot cook, then you are hostage to the supermarkets and food manufacturers. I used to be able to only cook breakfast and simple pasta dishes and the rest of the time I ate ready meals or ate out. About 16 years ago, I decided to change this and went on a two-month Italian cooking course at La Cucina Caldesi in London. That is where I met the chef Giancarlo Caldesi who became a great friend. He, along with his wife and chef Katie, have helped with the recipes in this book. I have always loved food and that first cooking class made me fall in love with cooking too, so much so that I have been on over 15 other cooking courses since! Perhaps you would also enjoy going on a cooking course to give you more confidence in the kitchen? Saying this, all the recipes in this book are suitable for novices. We also have plenty of videos on our website rewardsproject.org with quick tips, for example, on how to cook the perfect pasta and how to tell if your poached eggs are ready.

Meal preparation

We have done some of the hard work for you over the next two weeks by putting together delicious, healthy and great tasting recipes that you can easily prepare. We chose these recipes to give you a varied diet that will keep you satiated. There is a mix of meat, fish and vegetarian dishes. We also looked at the common meals that contain sugar – like shop-bought pasta sauces and tomato ketchup and devised great tasting alternatives with no added sugar! We even included a few of our favourite desserts.

To spread the workload, you can cook in larger batches e.g. our granola and our tomato sauce recipes can be cooked and then used throughout the week. We have indicated where you can freeze recipes and how long they will keep for in the fridge. For lunches, we recommend you prepare the night before to take into work, so stock up on Tupperware boxes or zip lock bags to store your food in. It will be much cheaper and more delicious than popping out for a sandwich.

Kicking sugar at work

We spend two-thirds of our lives at work, but have you ever thought about how healthy your office environment is? Clear out your desk and drawers of sweet treats just as you did at home. Get it out of your environment so you do not need to think about it. Initially replace your snacks with healthy ones. Nuts, oatcakes, Babybel cheese and fresh fruit. If you have access to a fridge then think hard-boiled eggs, cooked meats, chopped vegetables and hummus or nut butters. Over time, with three balanced meals a day you should feel full and satisfied and not need to snack. Snacking tends to be infectious. If no one else at your office is snacking then neither will you feel the need. It has been shown that the earlier you snack at work the more disinterested you are in your job. Perhaps an early warning sign that a colleague is going to resign is they open that snack drawer before everyone else!

Accountability

This challenge is going to be hard, especially if you have been eating lots of sugar and processed foods all your life. You will have help from this book and our Kick Sugar Facebook community, and I recommend enlisting your family and friends too. We advise setting up a private WhatsApp group for you to share recipes, photographs of your meals and generally encourage everyone on the journey.

Let everyone know you are doing the 14-day challenge, then there is less chance of you backing out or of someone at work offering you a doughnut. Ideally, get them to join you so you can share your successes. At Bow Lane Dental Group, we provided lunches for all the team that were on the challenge for two weeks, so all they needed to do was to cook breakfasts and dinners. Perhaps you can speak to your employer to see if they can do the same to invest in the health of their staff. Get them to sign our pledge (on page 186). We have a host of resources on our website for workplaces who want to do this challenge as a team.

Think about timing. I would avoid starting this challenge around birthdays, celebrations, holiday time, travelling and when you have a lot of evening events. It is impossible when you are not eating from your own kitchen to know what ingredients are in the foods. Over 70% of all supermarket goods have added sugar and we want to set you up for success. A study in 2010 found that nearly 90% of products on display at children's eye level in UK supermarkets are classed as unhealthy by the Food Standards Agency. In the last chapter, I'll give you tips on how to deal with these life events and still be low sugar.

Here are a few testimonials to inspire you!

"I gave up sugar in my tea after nearly 10 years!"
"Doing the challenge with a team of people helped with my motivation."
"I never normally eat fruit – but ate it more regularly on the challenge."
"With the group support I said no to cake and alcohol – even on my birthday!"
"Having a group chat to show each other our low-sugar dinners really helped."
"Great to try different things as it gave me more inspiration for my lunches."

Healthy habits

Your morning routine will help set you up for the day and this 14-day challenge. The routine that works best for me is: Wake at 6am, have one large glass of water, meditate for 20 minutes, write in my journal and then have a shower in readiness for the day. Your body likes routine and starting the day looking at social media on your phone just sets you up for depression! I like to be more proactive and focus first on the important things rather than get sucked into the urgent things, which often occur as soon as you turn your phone on. Perhaps you can use these 14 days to help set your body up with more healthy habits too.

FALSE BELIEFS

• COOKING IS HARD WORK!
Cooking can be easy and fun. Start off with simple dishes. Try something new each week. Your improved health should be the best motivation to experiment with more new dishes.

• RAW CARROTS ARE MORE NUTRITIOUS THAN COOKED
Some vegetables, carrots included, release more of their nutrients when they are cooked.

• AVOID EGGS BECAUSE OF HIGH CHOLESTEROL
While eggs are high in cholesterol they do not have a significant effect on blood cholesterol, whereas meat protein can be high in saturated fat, which will raise your blood cholesterol.

TOP TIPS

- Join our Facebook group, Kick Sugar.
- Buy all the ingredients you need for the challenge just before you start. The more you have invested in this experience the more likely you are going to succeed.
- Do not go shopping when you are hungry – you end up buying more than you want and are more likely to be tempted by processed packaged foods.
- Practising mindfulness has helped a lot of our patients get through any tough periods in this challenge.
- Try and notice your feelings throughout the day. When you are off the sugar roller-coaster you will be more aware of your feelings. Just listen to your body, acknowledge the feelings and move on. A good book to read about how the mind works is Michael Neil's *Supercoach*.

WEEK ONE

RECIPES

BREAKFASTS

Scrambled eggs with spinach and
   tomato
Poached eggs with smoked salmon
   and asparagus
Cacao quinoa porridge
Crunchy granola
Fruit and yoghurt sundae jars
Blueberry and oat pancakes
Savoury smoothie

LUNCHES

Speedy tomato sauce
Courgetti with tomato sauce
Chicken Caesar salad
Mexican prawn and avocado salad
Halloumi and spinach salad
Green omelette
Spicy squash and sage soup
Tuna poke bowl

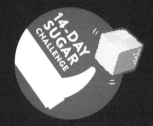

DINNERS

Pan-fried sole in caper and parsley
   butter with pearl barley
Thai green chicken curry
Chilli con carne with cauliflower rice
Spicy beef and broccoli stir-fry
Tuna pasta bake
Easy vegetable curry
Lemongrass and ginger salmon with
   Asian salad

CONDIMENTS

Homemade roasted tomato ketchup

DESSERTS

Coconut rice pudding with berry jam
Pear and apple crumble
Chocolate cake

Scrambled eggs with spinach and tomato v

Level	Prep time	Cook time	Days in fridge	Freeze
Easy	5 minutes	8 minutes	1	No

Serves 2

This is one of our favourite breakfast recipes as it is so quick and easy! If you don't have spinach, you can use kale or Swiss chard instead. We also sometimes finish this dish with a sprinkling of nuts or pumpkin seeds for added crunch and a nutrient boost.

1 tbsp unsalted butter
100g cherry tomatoes, halved
80g baby spinach
4 free-range eggs, lightly beaten
salt and freshly ground black pepper

1. Put the butter into a medium, non-stick saucepan over a medium heat. Add the tomatoes and a pinch of salt and cook for 3–4 minutes until soft.

2. Add the baby spinach, cover the pan with a lid and cook for a couple of minutes until wilted. Remove the lid, increase the heat and cook for a minute more to let excess water evaporate.

3. Lower the heat again to medium, add the eggs to the pan and cook for 1–2 minutes, stirring gently, until they are just set. Season with black pepper and serve.

Per serving					
Carbs	of which sugars	Protein	Fat	Fibre	Kcal
1.9g	1.8g	16g	17g	2.9g	232kcal

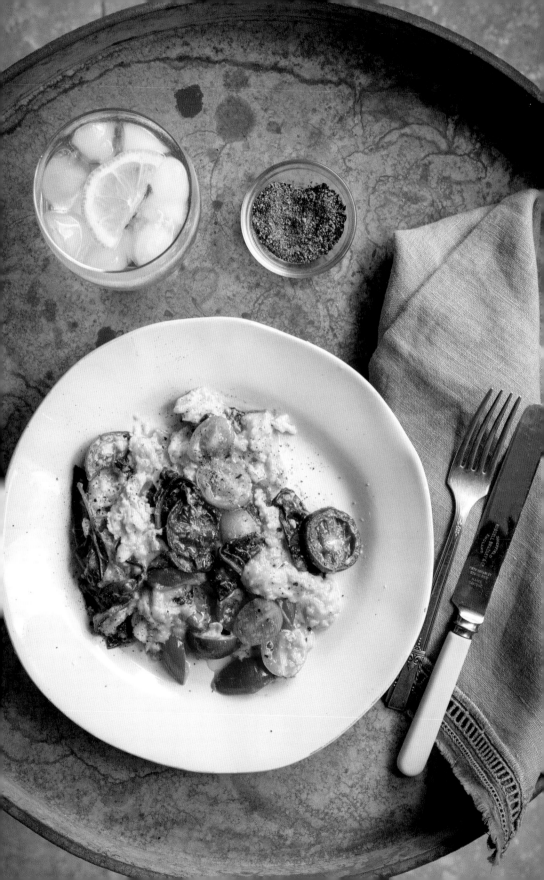

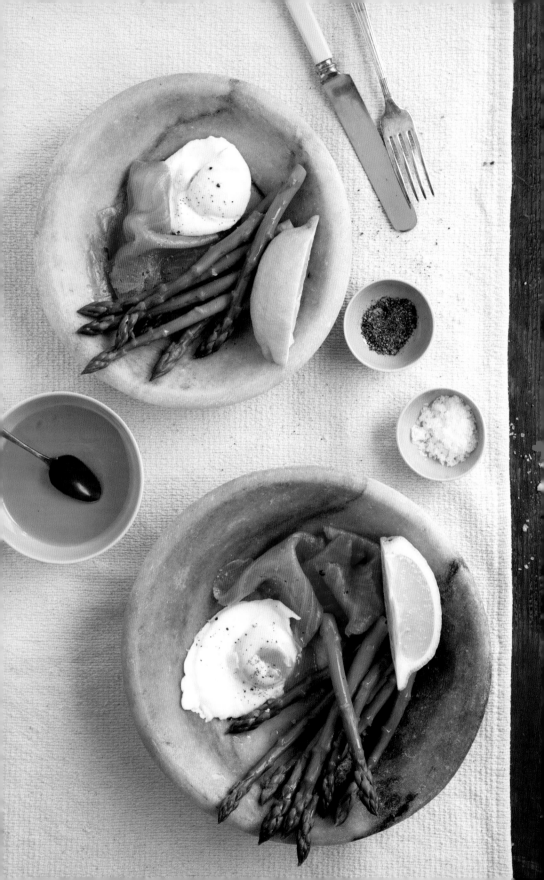

Poached eggs with smoked salmon and asparagus

Level	Prep time	Cook time	Days in fridge	Freeze
Moderate	2 minutes	5 minutes	I	No

Serves 2

Poached eggs are often messed up, but they are actually really simple to cook when you follow the right method. There is no need to stir the water as some people think, and it is best to boil the water initially and then reduce to a simmer. Cracking the eggs into coffee cups before adding to the water also helps them to keep their shape. When choosing smoked salmon, check for any added ingredients, such as extra salt or sugar. The smoking process naturally adds plenty of flavour, so the healthier option is to buy smoked salmon with no added extras.

100g smoked salmon
250g asparagus, woody ends removed
2 large free-range eggs
½ lemon, cut into quarters
salt and freshly ground black pepper

1. Arrange the smoked salmon on two serving plates.

2. Bring a large saucepan of salted water to the boil. Add the asparagus and cook for 2 minutes, then remove with a slotted spoon and drain well. Keep warm while you poach the eggs.

3. Keep the water simmering in the same pan that you cooked the asparagus in. Crack each egg into a coffee cup and then gently slide them into the simmering water. Simmer gently for 2–3 minutes for soft yolks.

4. Use a slotted spoon to lift the eggs from the water (you can gently poke the yolk with your finger to check the firmness) and drain on kitchen paper.

5. Serve the warm asparagus alongside the smoked salmon and poached eggs with a wedge of lemon and a twist of black pepper.

Per serving					
Carbs	of which sugars	Protein	Fat	Fibre	Kcal
3.5g	3.2g	23g	11g	3.3g	217kcal

Cacao quinoa porridge Ⓥ

Level	Prep time	Cook time	Days in fridge	Freeze
Easy	5 minutes	15–20 minutes	3	No

Serves 2

This recipe has one of the highest sugar contents because of the banana. In some low carbohydrate communities, the banana is evil! But I bet you didn't know that the type of carbohydrate found in each banana depends on its ripeness. Green or less ripe bananas contain less sugar and more resistant starch, so affect your blood sugar levels less. If you are not a diabetic, then they are fine in moderation.

1½ tbsp cacao powder
350ml full-fat dairy or nut milk
100g raw quinoa, rinsed
1 large banana, peeled and mashed
grated zest of 1 orange
2 tbsp chopped roasted hazelnuts

1. Mix the cacao powder with 50ml cold water in a jug to make a paste, then stir in the milk until smooth.

2. Pour the cacao milk into a small saucepan, add the quinoa and mashed banana and mix.

3. Bring to the boil, then reduce the heat, cover the pan and simmer gently for 10–15 minutes, stirring frequently, until the quinoa is tender.

4. Portion into bowls and sprinkle with orange zest and chopped roasted hazelnuts to serve.

Per serving					
Carbs	of which sugars	Protein	Fat	Fibre	Kcal
45g	20g	16g	13g	9.1g	381kcal

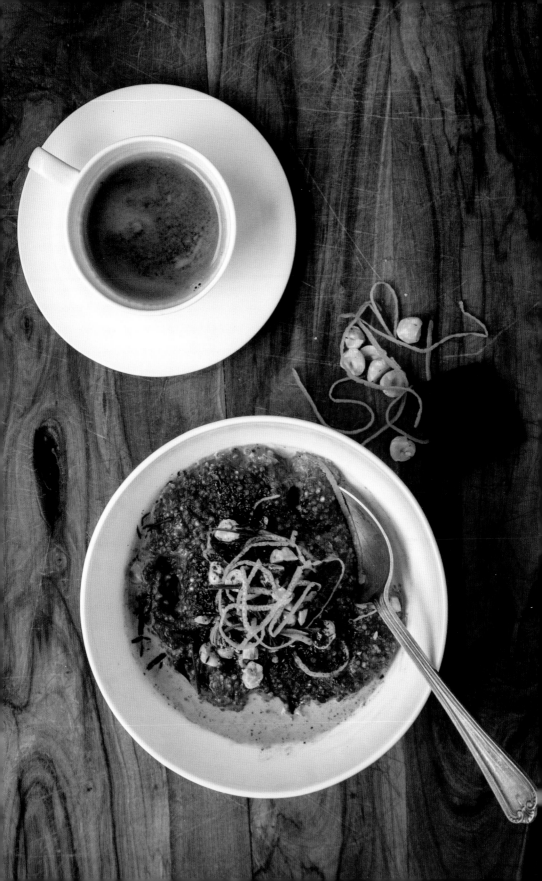

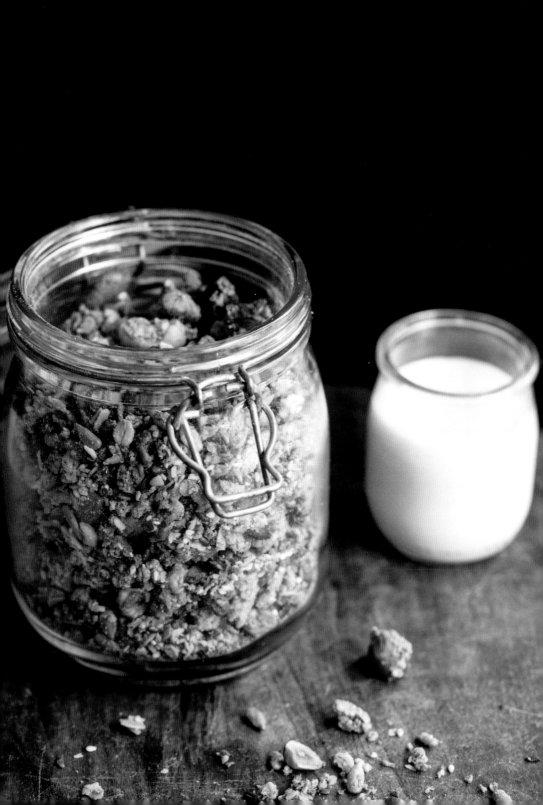

Crunchy granola v

Level	Prep time	Cook time	Days in storage	Freeze
Easy	10 minutes	30 minutes	28	No

Makes 500g (10 x 50g servings)

This recipe is great for using up any nuts you have in your kitchen cupboards. In my family, it rarely lasts a month, as everyone picks at it. We think it tastes great without the apple, but if you like your granola in clumps, then using a puréed apple or juice helps to bind it together more.

100g porridge oats
100g ground almonds
100g mixed nuts (pecans, cashews or
   almonds, etc.)
100g mixed seeds (pumpkin, flaxseeds or
   sunflower, etc.)
50g desiccated coconut or dried coconut chips
   (unsweetened)
1 tbsp ground cinnamon
1 egg white
pinch of salt
1 tbsp vanilla extract
60g coconut oil, melted
25ml apple juice (or 1 peeled and cored eating
   apple puréed raw with a splash of water)

1. Preheat the oven to 150°C fan/170°C/ gas mark 4 and line a large baking tray with baking paper.

2. Mix all the dry ingredients together in a large bowl (oats, nuts, seeds, coconut and cinnamon) and set aside.

3. Place the egg white, salt and vanilla extract in a separate bowl and whisk together by hand until frothy. Add to the bowl of dry ingredients with the melted coconut oil and apple juice (or purée) and mix thoroughly.

4. Tip onto the lined baking tray and spread out evenly. Bake in the oven for 30 minutes, stirring at intervals, until pale golden in colour.

5. Remove from the oven and leave to cool completely on the tray before serving and/or transferring to a large, clean airtight jar.

Per serving

Carbs	of which sugars	Protein	Fat	Fibre	Kcal
8.6g	1.4g	6.1g	21g	4.3g	260kcal

Fruit and yoghurt sundae jars v

Level	Prep time	Days in fridge	Freeze
Easy	5 minutes	3	No

Serves 2

Prepare this in a jam jar with a lid if you need a breakfast to go.

100g Crunchy Granola (see page 87)
150g natural Greek yoghurt (or unsweetened non-dairy yoghurt)
150g fresh mixed berries (blueberries, raspberries, strawberries, etc.)
1 tbsp chia seeds

Layer the crunchy granola, yoghurt and berries in glass sundae dishes or bowls, top with chia seeds and enjoy!

Per serving					
Carbs	of which sugars	Protein	Fat	Fibre	Kcal
17g	9.3g	12g	31g	8.3g	415kcal

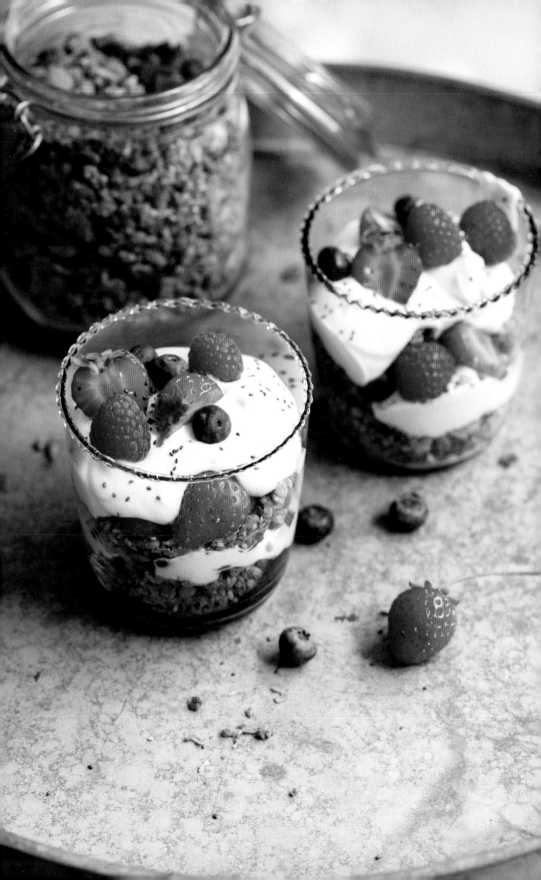

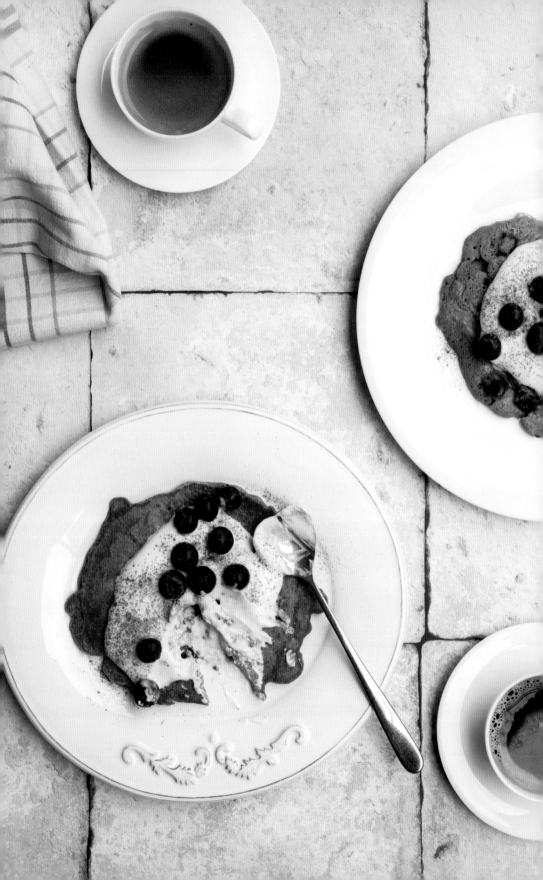

Blueberry and oat pancakes v

Level	Prep time	Cook time	Days in fridge	Freeze
Moderate	10 minutes	5 minutes	2	Yes

Serves 2

If you can't get your hands on wholemeal self-raising flour for these American-style pancakes, you can make your own by mixing 75g wholemeal flour with ½ tsp baking powder.

50g porridge oats
75g wholemeal self-raising flour
1 tsp ground cinnamon, plus extra for sprinkling (optional)
100ml full-fat milk
1 egg, lightly beaten
130g fresh blueberries, halved, plus extra whole blueberries to decorate
2–3 tbsp coconut oil
60g natural Greek yoghurt (or unsweetened non-dairy yoghurt), to serve

1. Put the dry ingredients (oats, flour and cinnamon) in a blender and pulse to evenly combine. Add the milk, egg and 60ml water and pulse again until combined into a batter. Stir in the halved blueberries and then let the batter rest for 5 minutes.

2. Put a large, non-stick frying pan over a medium-high heat. Add the coconut oil to the pan and let it melt, tilting the pan to coat the base. Place 3 tbsp of batter into the pan (one for each pancake).

3. Cook for about 1–2 minutes until you begin to see bubbles form in the middle of each pancake, then flip over and cook on the other side for about 30 seconds or until browned. Remove to a plate and keep warm.

4. Repeat the cooking process with the remaining batter and serve the pancakes with yoghurt and extra whole blueberries. Sprinkle with extra cinnamon to finish, if you like.

Per serving					
Carbs	of which sugars	Protein	Fat	Fibre	Kcal
49g	10g	16g	19g	4g	445kcal

Savoury smoothie (V)

Level	Prep time	Days in fridge	Freeze
Easy	5 minutes	3	Yes

Serves 2

This is really easy to make, and the avocado gives it a delicious creamy texture.

½ cucumber, roughly chopped
1 small avocado, halved, peeled and stoned
50g fennel or 1 celery stalk, roughly chopped, plus extra to decorate (optional)
1 sprig mint, leaves picked and stalks discarded, plus a sprig to decorate (optional)
1 tbsp unsweetened almond butter
100ml water or coconut water

Place all of the ingredients into a blender and blitz until smooth. Pour into glasses to serve. Decorate with an extra celery stalk and mint sprig, if you like.

Photo opposite shows the savoury smoothie (behind) with the sweet smoothie from page 146

Per serving (without garnish)

Carbs	of which sugars	Protein	Fat	Fibre	Kcal
2.7g	1.2g	3.6g	19g	5.8g	209kcal

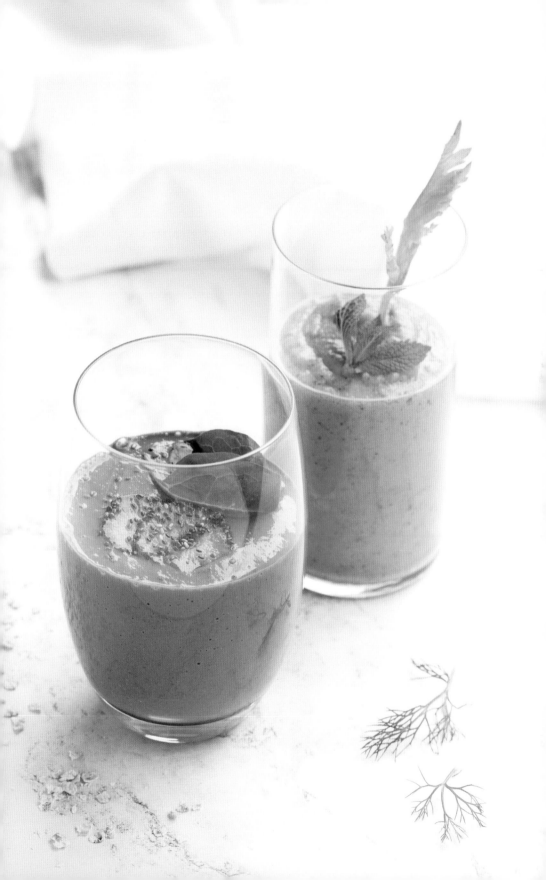

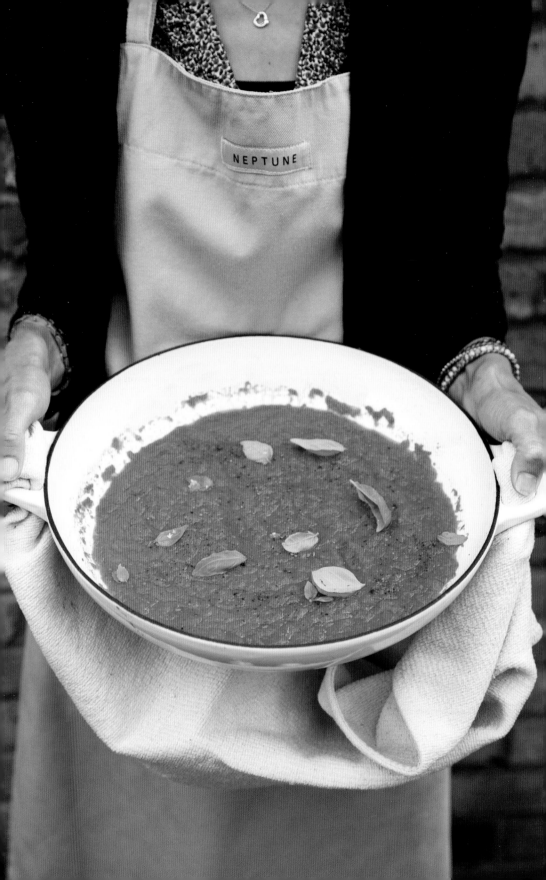

Speedy tomato sauce v

Level	Prep time	Cook time	Days in fridge	Freeze
Easy	5 minutes	30 minutes	7	Yes

Makes approx. 700g

This is such a versatile sauce. In this book, we use it in the Meatballs with Beans and Cheese (see page 166), One-pot Sausage Casserole (see page 162) and with courgetti (see page 96). This recipe makes a large batch that will be enough to make all of these meals. It can be stored in an airtight container and kept in the fridge for up to 1 week, or frozen for up to 2 months.

3 tbsp olive oil
2 red onions, very finely chopped
3 garlic cloves, finely grated
2 x 400g tins whole plum tomatoes
15g fresh basil leaves, torn
salt and freshly ground black pepper

1. Put the olive oil into a large saucepan over a medium heat. Add the red onions and garlic and season with salt and pepper. Cook for 5–8 minutes, stirring occasionally to avoid browning, until the onions are soft, translucent and sweet.

2. Add the tomatoes to the pan, stir, cover with a lid and simmer gently for 20 minutes.

3. Stir in the torn basil leaves and add more seasoning to taste if needed. Blitz with a hand-held stick blender if you like a smoother sauce.

4. Serve hot or leave to cool before storing in the fridge.

Per serving (100g)					
Carbs	of which sugars	Protein	Fat	Fibre	Kcal
4g	3.3g	0.7g	3.3g	0.9g	53kcal

Courgetti with tomato sauce

Level	Prep time	Cook time	Days in fridge	Freeze
Easy	5 minutes	8 minutes	5	No

Serves 2

Here is a low carbohydrate version of spaghetti with tomato sauce, which is much faster to cook! You could also serve courgetti with homemade Bolognese sauce or the pesto sauce (see page 157). This dish also works cold if you need a portable lunch, just mix the cold sauce with the raw courgetti and garnish.

30g pine nuts
200g Speedy Tomato Sauce (see page 95)
2 courgettes, spiralised or ribbons made with a peeler
30g Parmesan cheese (or vegetarian hard cheese alternative), grated
freshly ground black pepper

1. Place a small frying pan over a medium heat. Add the pine nuts and toast for 2–3 minutes until golden, shaking the pan occasionally to make sure they don't burn. Set aside.

2. Place the tomato sauce in a large saucepan over a medium heat and warm through until steaming hot. Remove the pan from the heat and stir in the courgetti.

3. Serve topped with grated Parmesan, the toasted pine nuts and plenty of black pepper.

Per serving

Carbs	of which sugars	Protein	Fat	Fibre	Kcal
8.4g	7.4g	12g	19g	5.4g	265kcal

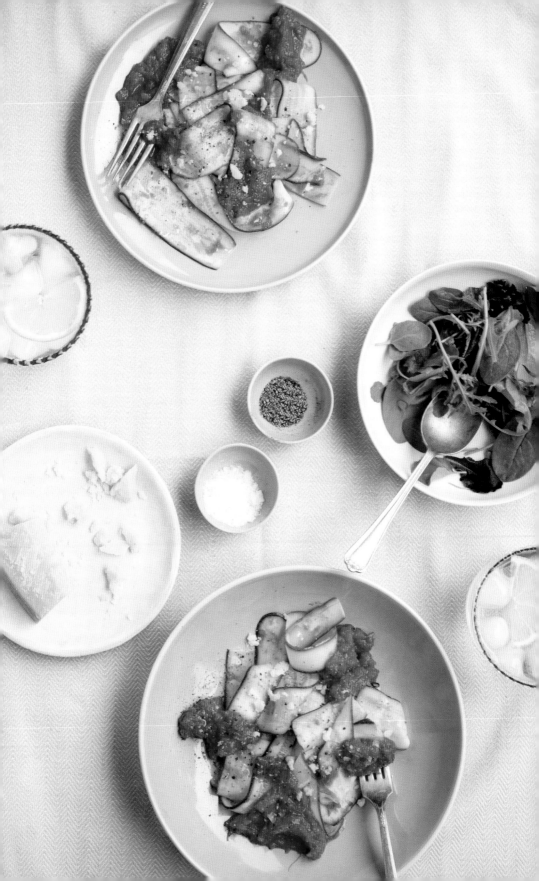

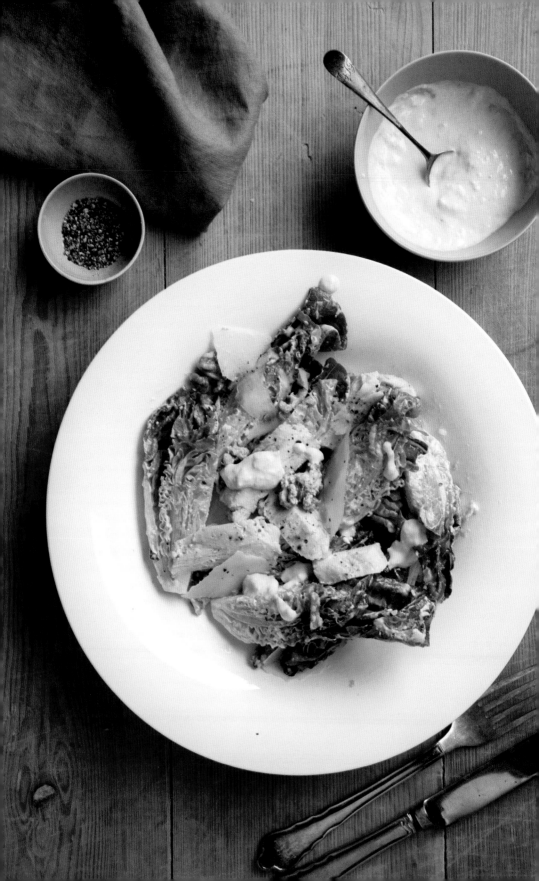

Chicken Caesar salad

Level	Prep time	Cook time	Days in fridge	Freeze
Easy	15 minutes	10 minutes	5	No

Serves 2

There is often hidden sugar in ready-cooked chicken so it's always best to cook your own from scratch – and it tastes so much better too! This method of butterflying the chicken first is useful as it speeds up the cooking time.

2 chicken breasts
1 tbsp olive oil
1 lettuce, thickly sliced (romaine, cos, little gem or ruby gem, etc.)
20g walnuts
15g Parmesan cheese, grated
salt and freshly ground black pepper

For the dressing
1 small garlic clove, finely chopped
2 tinned anchovies, very finely chopped
freshly squeezed juice of ½ lemon
1 tsp Dijon mustard
60g natural Greek yoghurt
15g Parmesan cheese, grated

1. First, butterfly the chicken breasts (this will help them to cook more quickly and evenly). To do this, place the chicken onto a chopping board and use a sharp knife to cut horizontally into each breast down the side, taking care not to cut all the way through. Open out the butterflied chicken and season both sides with salt and pepper.

2. Put the olive oil into a large frying pan over a medium heat. Add the opened-out chicken breasts and cook for 3 minutes. Turn the chicken over and cover the pan with a lid. Turn the heat to low and cook for 5 more minutes until cooked through. Switch off the heat and rest, covered, for 5 minutes.

3. Pull the chicken into bite-size chunks in the pan and leave it to soak up all of the cooking juices while you make the dressing.

4. Combine all the dressing ingredients in a bowl, season with black pepper and mix together thoroughly.

5. To assemble the salad, divide the lettuce slices and walnuts between serving bowls. Drizzle over the dressing and toss together with the leaves and nuts. Top each salad with the warm cooked chicken and scatter with grated Parmesan to finish.

Per serving

Carbs	of which sugars	Protein	Fat	Fibre	Kcal
2.8g	2.5g	50g	18g	1.2g	379kcal

Mexican prawn and avocado salad

Level	Prep time	Days in fridge	Freeze
Easy	5 minutes	I	No

Serves 2

This is a tasty and really speedy lunch; just make sure the tortilla chips you buy are good quality and don't have added glucose syrup and sugar or MSG (monosodium glutamate). If you want to reduce the carb content, then replace the tortilla chips with mixed seeds.

I large avocado, halved, peeled and stoned
freshly squeezed juice of I lime
50g cherry tomatoes, quartered
I red chilli, sliced
handful of fresh coriander, chopped
½ x 400g tin black beans, drained and rinsed
50g rocket or baby spinach leaves
200g cooked peeled prawns
80g salted tortilla chips

1. Cut the avocado into chunks and place in a bowl with the lime juice, cherry tomatoes, chilli, coriander and black beans. Mix together well.

2. Arrange the rocket or spinach leaves on serving plates and dollop over the avocado mixture. Top the salads with cooked prawns and roughly break up and scatter the tortilla chips over the top to finish.

Per serving

Carbs	of which sugars	Protein	Fat	Fibre	Kcal
36g	4.3g	25g	25g	I Ig	492kcal

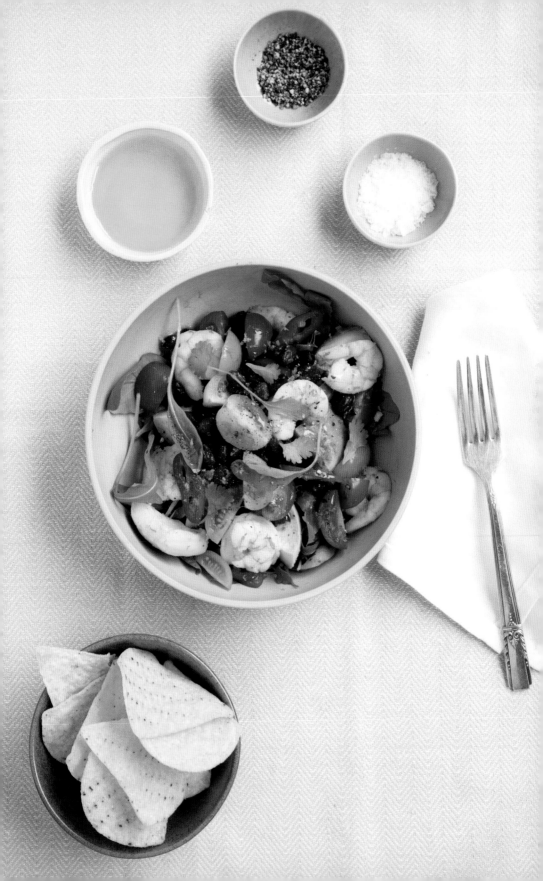

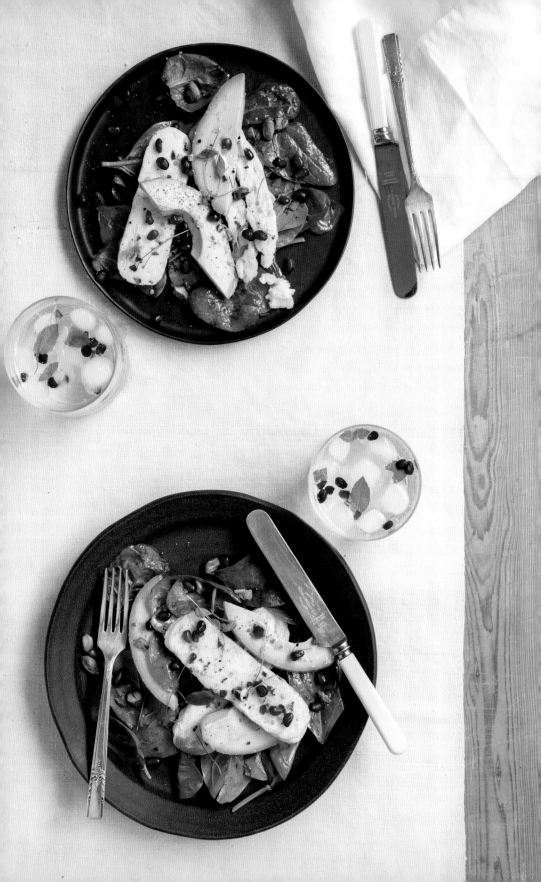

Halloumi and spinach salad v

Level	Prep time	Cook time	Days in fridge	Freeze
Easy	10 minutes	5 minutes	5	No

Serves 2

The saltiness of the halloumi goes well with the fresh spinach in this salad, and the pomegranate gives it a sweet taste too. You can add raw sugar snap peas or steamed asparagus for extra greens, if you like. Halloumi starts to harden as it cools so eat immediately.

For the dressing
3 tbsp extra virgin olive oil
1 tbsp wholegrain mustard
grated zest and freshly squeezed juice
   of ½ lemon
salt and freshly ground black pepper

For the salad
80g baby spinach
1 large avocado, peeled, stoned and sliced
30g pistachio nuts, gently crushed
65g pomegranate seeds (about half a medium
   pomegranate)
225g halloumi, cut into slices
1 tsp dried chilli flakes
pinch of cumin seeds

1. First, place all the dressing ingredients into a jam jar, put the lid on and shake well, adding salt and black pepper to taste. If you don't have a jam jar, then just whisk the ingredients together in a small bowl.

2. Place the spinach, avocado, pistachio nuts and pomegranate seeds into a large bowl. Pour over the dressing and toss together. Set aside.

3. Sprinkle the halloumi slices evenly with the dried chilli flakes and cumin seeds.

4. Place a large, shallow non-stick frying pan over a high heat. Add the halloumi and dry-fry for a couple of minutes, then turn over and cook for another 2 minutes until brown on both sides.

5. Arrange the salad on serving plates and top with the fried halloumi.

Per serving					
Carbs	of which sugars	Protein	Fat	Fibre	Kcal
9.7g	7.5g	34g	72g	7g	844kcal

Green omelette v

Level	Prep time	Cook time	Days in fridge	Freeze
Easy	5 minutes	10 minutes	1	No

Serves 1

We love the versatility of omelettes. Depending on the range of ingredients used they can be breakfast, lunch or dinner. The size of your frying pan is key, around 22cm is ideal for a 3- or 4-egg omelette. Too big and your omelette will overcook and be too thin. An omelette goes on cooking even on the plate, so be sure to serve it immediately.

20g unsalted butter
1 red onion, sliced into semi-circles
100g spinach
4 medium free-range eggs, lightly beaten (room temperature)
70g feta cheese
salt and freshly ground black pepper

1. Put the butter in a 22cm frying pan over a medium heat. Add the red onion and sauté. When it is still slightly crunchy, add the spinach, cover the pan with a lid and cook for about 2 minutes to wilt. Remove the spinach and onions from the pan and set aside.

2. Add the eggs to the same pan, then cook without stirring over a medium heat for about 1 minute 30 seconds or until almost set. Add the cooked onion and spinach and crumble in the feta on one side of the omelette so you can fold it over.

3. After another 30 seconds, flip the omelette over to cook on the other side.

4. Cook for 2 more minutes, then season with salt and black pepper and fold to serve.

Per serving					
Carbs	of which sugars	Protein	Fat	Fibre	Kcal
6.3g	4.5g	22g	26g	3g	352kcal

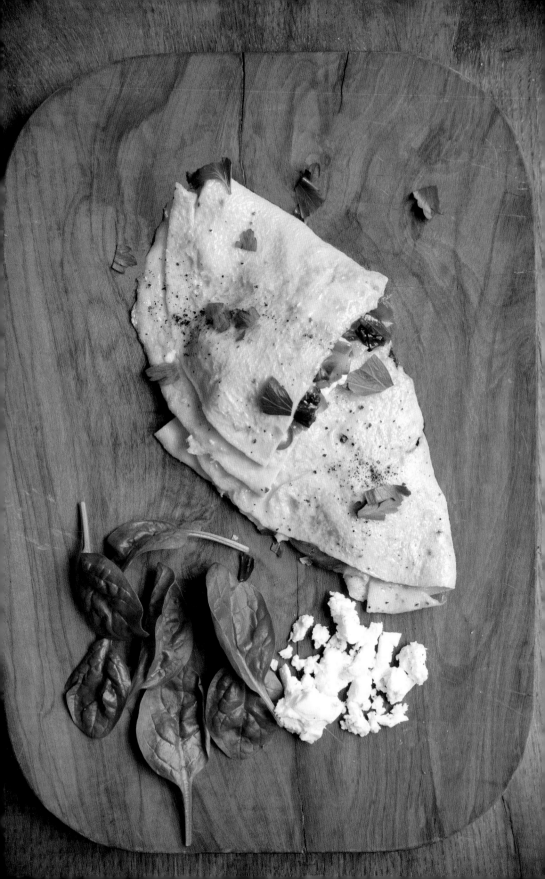

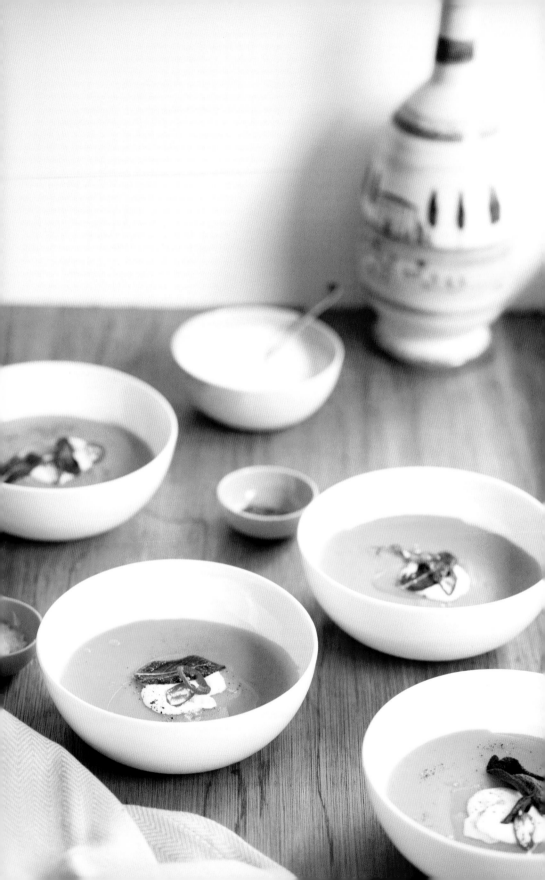

Spicy squash and sage soup

Level	Prep time	Cook time	Days in fridge	Freeze
Easy	15 minutes	20–25 minutes	7	Yes

Serves 2

This is a wonderful warming soup with a creamy taste despite not using cream. The earthy, musty flavour of the sage helps to take the soup to another level. Sage works just as well to enhance a mushroom or minestrone soup. Fry a few extra leaves as they are delicious as a snack.

3 tbsp olive oil
200g butternut squash, peeled, deseeded and cut into 1cm cubes (prepared weight)
1 red onion, roughly chopped
1 large garlic clove, roughly chopped
1 large red chilli, stalk removed, quartered, plus extra to serve
1 tsp cumin seeds
120g dried red lentils
650ml hot water or vegetable or chicken stock
4 fresh sage leaves
salt and freshly ground black pepper
crème fraîche, to serve (optional)

1. Place a large saucepan over a medium heat and add 2 tbsp of the oil. Add the butternut squash, red onion, garlic, chilli and cumin seeds and cook for about 5–7 minutes until softened.

2. Add the red lentils and hot water or stock and bring to the boil, then reduce the heat, cover with a lid and simmer for 15–20 minutes.

3. Season the soup with salt and black pepper and use a hand-held stick blender or transfer carefully to a blender and blitz until smooth.

Return the soup to the pan over a low heat to keep warm until ready to serve.

4. Heat the remaining 1 tbsp oil in a small frying pan and add the sage leaves. Fry for around a minute until crisp, taking care that they don't burn.

5. Pour the soup into two warmed bowls and add the crispy sage leaves. Serve topped with crème fraîche, extra sliced chilli and more black pepper, if you like.

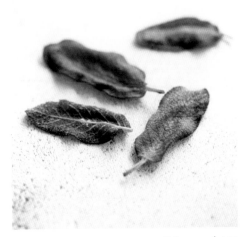

Crispy sage leaves

Per serving (based on water rather than stock option; crème fraîche not included)					
Carbs	of which sugars	Protein	Fat	Fibre	Kcal
47g	10g	17g	20g	6.5g	453kcal

Tuna poke bowl

Level	Prep time	Cook time	Days in fridge	Freeze
Easy	15 minutes	20 minutes	1	No

Serves 2

We love the freshness of this bowl and its delicate flavours. You could substitute the tuna for salmon if you prefer. Whichever you choose, try and use the freshest fish (sushi grade is best) and refrigerate it as soon as you can. Ideally consume it within one day to be safe.

100g brown basmati rice, rinsed thoroughly
2 tbsp soy sauce
1 tbsp sesame oil
1 tbsp rice vinegar
1 lime
½ tsp peeled and grated fresh ginger
200g very fresh skinless tuna or salmon, cut into small cubes
1 avocado, peeled, stoned and cut into cubes
2 spring onions, finely sliced
¼ red cabbage, very finely shredded
1 carrot, peeled and grated
few sprigs fresh coriander
1 tsp white or black sesame seeds

1. Place the rice in a small saucepan with 250ml water and bring to the boil. Lower the heat, cover and simmer gently for about 20–25 minutes or according to the packet instructions. All the water should have been absorbed when the rice is cooked. Spread the rice out on a large plate to let it cool as quickly as possible.

2. Meanwhile, combine the soy sauce, sesame oil, rice vinegar, juice of half the lime (keep the other half for garnish), and ginger in a mixing bowl. Add the tuna or salmon cubes, avocado and spring onions and mix to combine.

3. In a separate bowl, mix together the red cabbage and carrot to combine.

4. To assemble the poke bowls, place the cooled rice into two serving bowls. Add the tuna/salmon mixture next to it, the red cabbage and carrot mixture, coriander and a sprinkle of sesame seeds. Cut the remaining lime half into slices and serve alongside the poke for squeezing over.

5. For the best taste, refrigerate for 15 minutes before eating.

Per serving					
Carbs	of which sugars	Protein	Fat	Fibre	Kcal
47g	7.4g	34g	22g	8g	546kcal

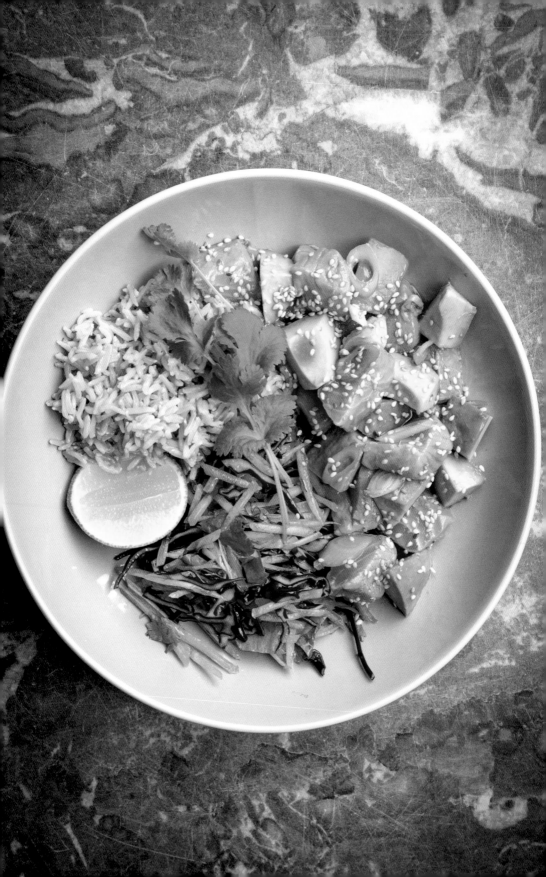

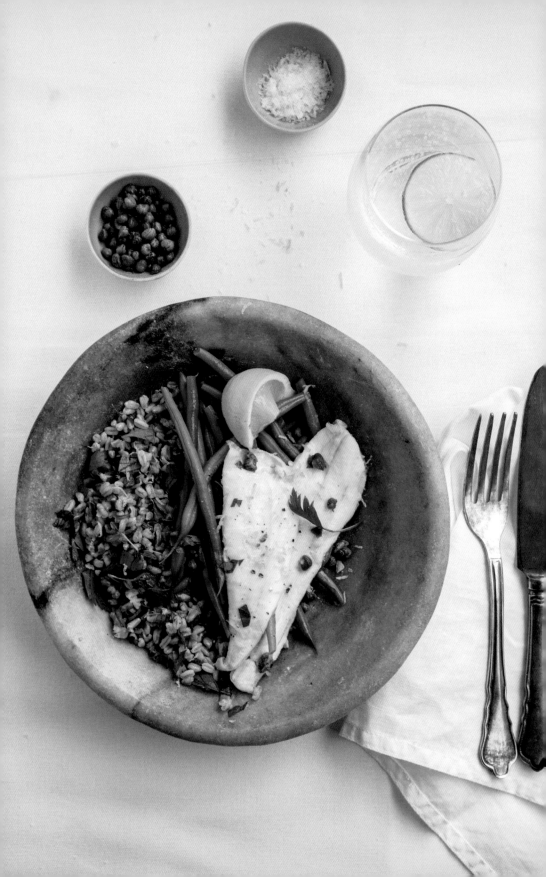

Pan-fried sole in caper and parsley butter with pearl barley

Level	Prep time	Cook time	Days in fridge	Freeze
Moderate	5 minutes	30 minutes	1	No

Serves 2

You can do this recipe with any flat fish such as plaice, megrim sole and dover sole, but lemon sole is good value for money and easier to get hold of at most supermarkets or fishmongers. You can accompany it with 350g cooked new potatoes if you don't fancy grains.

120g pearl barley, faro or other whole grain wheat, well rinsed
250g lemon sole or dover sole fillets, with or without skin
150g green beans
20g unsalted butter
½ tbsp olive oil
3 tbsp capers, drained
few sprigs parsley, leaves picked and finely chopped
salt and freshly ground black pepper
lemon wedges, to serve

1. Put the pearl barley or whole grain wheat in a large saucepan with 600ml water. Bring to the boil, then lower the heat and simmer for 30 minutes until tender (see packet instructions if not using pearl barley).

2. Meanwhile, place the fish fillets onto some kitchen paper and pat dry with some more kitchen paper. Season the fish with salt and black pepper. Set aside for a moment.

3. Bring another small saucepan of water to the boil. Add the green beans and simmer for about 5 minutes until just tender. Drain and then keep them warm until needed.

4. In a large, non-stick frying pan, melt the butter with the oil over a low heat. Add the fish fillets (skin-side-down if using skin-on) and cook for 2 minutes. Very gently turn the fillets over and cook for another 2 minutes on the other side or until the fish is cooked through.

5. Turn off the heat, then add the capers and chopped parsley leaves to the pan to warm through in the butter for a moment.

6. Drain the pearl barley when it's cooked and put onto serving plates alongside the fish and green beans. Drizzle with the caper and parsley butter from the pan and serve with lemon wedges for squeezing over.

Per serving (based on pearl barley)					
Carbs	of which sugars	Protein	Fat	Fibre	Kcal
48g	1.8g	28g	14g	2.8g	431kcal

Thai green chicken curry

Level	Prep time	Cook time	Days in fridge	Freeze
Advanced	15 minutes	20–25 minutes	2	Yes

Serves 2

This is a classic curry with a rich and aromatic flavour. You could make a double batch of the paste and store it in the fridge in a sterilised jar covered with a layer of oil for up to a month. Swapping the chicken for frozen prawns or fish and using frozen green beans, peas or spinach is a great way to ensure you always have a fresh meal on hand when time is short. If you want to reduce the GI further you can swap the brown rice for a delicious cauliflower rice (see page 115). This rice is fast to make with a food processor and ready in just five minutes.

For the curry paste
2 garlic cloves, peeled
3cm fresh ginger, peeled and roughly chopped
10g fresh coriander, roughly chopped
1 tbsp ground cumin
1–3 red chillies (to taste), stalks removed, sliced
1 lemongrass stalk, outer skin removed,
   chopped in half lengthways
2 fresh or dried kaffir lime leaves
1–2 tbsp soy sauce
1 tbsp olive oil

For the curry
2 tbsp coconut oil
2 free-range chicken breasts, cut into strips
1 red pepper, deseeded and cut into strips
1 x 400g tin unsweetened coconut milk
125g sugar snap peas
salt and freshly ground black pepper

To serve
120g brown basmati rice, rinsed thoroughly
10g fresh coriander, roughly chopped

1. Place all the curry paste ingredients into a food processor or mini chopper and pulse to form a paste. Scrape into a bowl and set aside.

2. Place the rice into a small saucepan with 300ml water. Bring to the boil, then lower the heat, cover with a lid and simmer gently for about 20–25 minutes or according the packet instructions until the water has been absorbed and the rice is cooked. Switch off the heat and keep the pan covered to keep the rice warm.

3. Meanwhile, melt the coconut oil in a large, heavy-based frying pan over a high heat. Season the chicken with salt and black pepper and add to the pan. Add the red pepper and stir-fry for a minute or two.

4. Stir in the curry paste and cook for 3–5 minutes.

5. Stir in the coconut milk and sugar snap peas and bring to a simmer for a final 2 minutes until the chicken is cooked through.

6. Scatter with fresh coriander and serve in warm bowls alongside the cooked basmati rice.

Per serving					
Carbs	of which sugars	Protein	Fat	Fibre	Kcal
62g	10g	43g	68g	3.2g	1043kcal

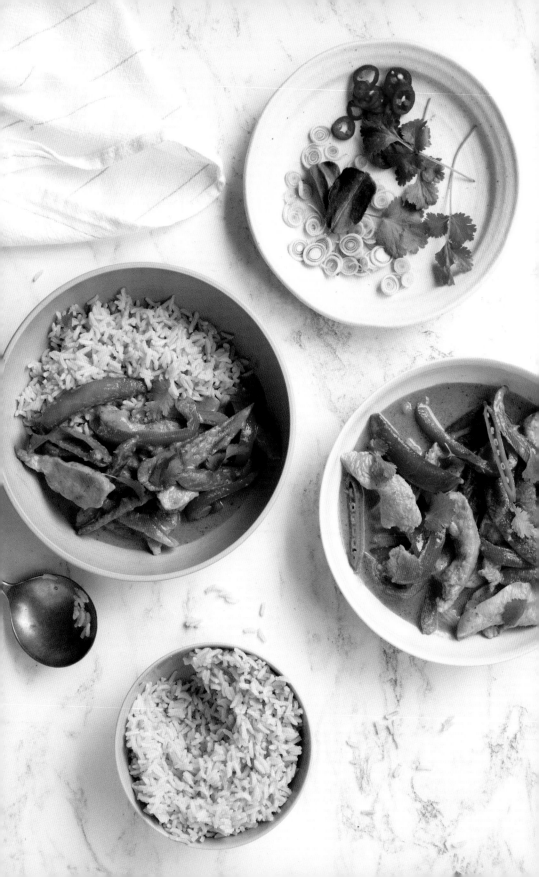

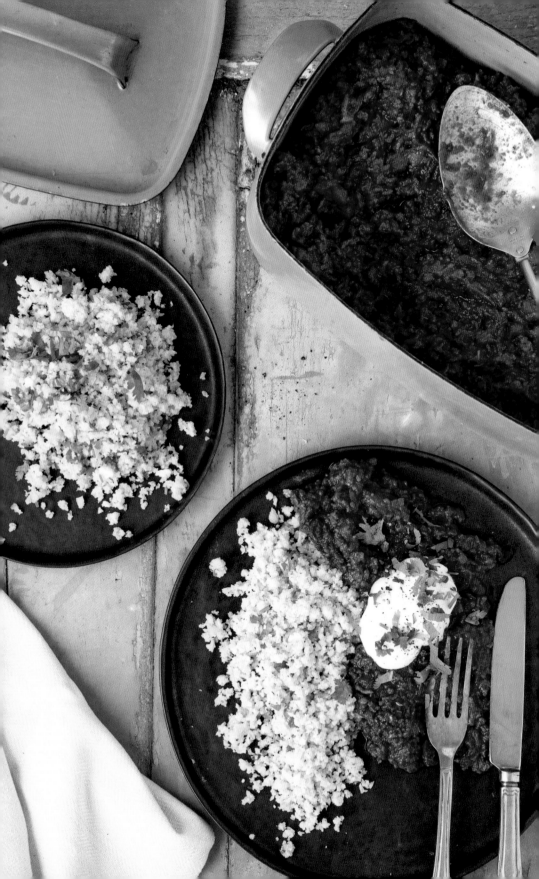

Chilli con carne with cauliflower rice

Level	Prep time	Cook time	Days in fridge	Freeze
Moderate	15 minutes	1–2 hours	2	Yes

Serves 4

For a meat-free alternative here, use 800g chestnut mushrooms instead of the minced beef. We mention simmering for 45 minutes, but the longer the cooking time the more tender the meat will be. Adding cacao powder at the end will bring a richness to the chilli, plus all the health benefits we talked about earlier.

For the chilli con carne
500g minced beef
2 tbsp olive oil
1 large onion, finely chopped
2 garlic cloves, grated
1 heaped tsp cumin seeds
½–1 tsp chilli powder (to taste)
1 tbsp tomato purée
125ml red wine
1 x 400g tin whole plum tomatoes
1 x 400g tin beans, drained (kidney beans, black beans, pinto beans, etc.)
1 tbsp cacao powder, plus extra to serve
salt and freshly ground black pepper
2 heaped tbsp natural Greek yoghurt, to serve

For the cauliflower rice
1 cauliflower (about 300g), quartered
2 tbsp olive oil
10g fresh coriander, finely chopped

1. Place a large, heavy-based frying pan over a medium heat and add the beef to dry-fry. Season well with salt and black pepper and mix as it cooks to break up the meat. Cook for about 8 minutes until the outside of the beef has browned.

2. Remove the beef with a spoon to a plate and add the olive oil to the pan. Add the onion, garlic and cumin seeds and fry for 5 minutes until softened.

3. Add the chilli powder and tomato purée. Return the meat to the pan and mix everything together. Turn the heat to high, add the red wine and let it bubble for a few minutes until mostly evaporated. Stir in the tinned tomatoes and beans.

4. Cover the pan and simmer over the lowest heat for a minimum of 45 minutes and a maximum of 2 hours, topping up with water if the pan dries out. Mix in the cacao powder 5 minutes before the end of the cooking time.

5. When you are nearly ready to serve the chilli, put the cauliflower in a food processor and blitz to a rice texture. Heat the olive oil in a separate large shallow frying pan and fry the cauliflower rice with a splash of water for 5 minutes. Season with salt and black pepper and mix in the coriander.

6. Serve the cauliflower rice with the chilli, a dollop of yoghurt and an extra sprinkling of cacao powder.

Per serving (based on 400g tinned kidney beans)

Carbs	of which sugars	Protein	Fat	Fibre	Kcal
62g	23g	78g	63g	28g	1233kcal

Spicy beef and broccoli stir-fry

Level	Prep time	Cook time	Days in fridge	Freeze
Moderate	10 minutes	12 minutes	3	Yes

Serves 2

The trick here is to get all the ingredients ready and to hand before you start cooking so that you can easily chuck them into the pan. Keep the pan really hot and keep the ingredients moving using tongs or by tossing them in the pan. If you are doubling the recipe, then make this in two batches so that the pan isn't overcrowded.

For the dressing
1 tsp dried chilli flakes
2 tbsp soy sauce
1 tbsp vinegar (cider or rice vinegar, etc.)

For the stir-fry
150g Tenderstem or normal broccoli, broken into small florets
1 red onion, very finely sliced
1 garlic clove, chopped
3cm fresh ginger, peeled and finely shredded into matchsticks
50g raw cashew nuts
2 x nests dried wholewheat noodles (200g)
4 tbsp groundnut oil
250g minute steak, cut into strips
6 sprigs fresh coriander, roughly torn
75g frozen peas
salt and freshly ground black pepper

1. Mix the dressing ingredients together in a small bowl and set aside.

2. Mix the broccoli, red onion, garlic, ginger and cashew nuts together in a bowl and set aside.

3. Bring a small saucepan of water to the boil and add the noodles. Switch off the heat and leave for 4 minutes. Drain, then rinse the noodles in cold water and drain well again. Place the noodles in a bowl and toss with 1 tbsp of the groundnut oil. Set aside.

4. Season the steak strips with a touch of salt and plenty of black pepper and place next to the hob. Get out the coriander and peas ready to use too.

5. To cook the stir-fry, heat a heavy-based frying pan or wok until searing hot, then add the remaining 3 tbsp groundnut oil. Immediately add the mixed vegetables and toss in the oil or use tongs to turn and stir-fry for 2–3 minutes.

6. Add the steak slices, frozen peas and coriander and toss through for 1–2 minutes until the peas are hot. We are looking for the steak to be slightly pink in the middle. Cook for longer if you prefer it cooked through.

7. Add the noodles and finally the dressing. Stir-fry for 1 minute longer, making sure all the ingredients are coated in the dressing. Remove from the heat and serve.

Per serving					
Carbs	of which sugars	Protein	Fat	Fibre	Kcal
44g	10g	47g	38g	9.5g	723kcal

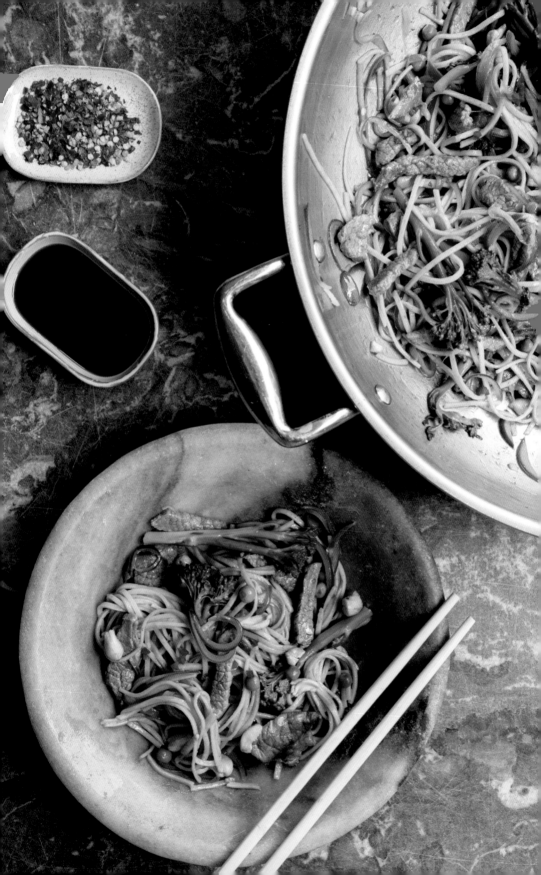

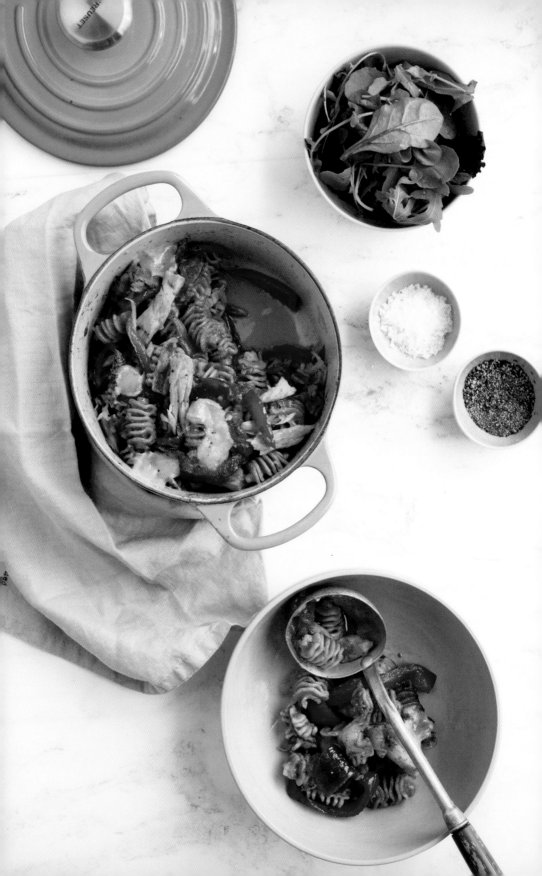

Tuna pasta bake

Level	Prep time	Cook time	Days in fridge	Freeze
Easy	10 minutes	35 minutes	3	No

Serves 2

Pasta bakes are very good for a midweek meal when you are in a hurry. They can be pre-assembled and then just put in the oven when you are almost ready to eat.

150g wholewheat dried pasta (Radiatori, penne, fusilli or farfalle, etc.)
1 x 200g tin tuna in olive oil
1 red onion, cut into 8 wedges
1 red pepper, deseeded and cut into strips
1 garlic clove, chopped
2 tsp tomato purée
1 x 400g tin whole plum tomatoes
50g Cheddar cheese, grated
few sprigs fresh parsley, finely chopped
salt and freshly ground black pepper

1. Bring a large saucepan of water to the boil. Add the pasta and simmer for 10 minutes or until al dente. Drain and set aside.

2. Preheat the oven to 200°C fan/220°C/ gas mark 7.

3. Place a large, heavy-based saucepan over a medium heat and add the oil from the tin of tuna, the red onion, red pepper, garlic and tomato purée and fry for 3–4 minutes.

4. Add the tuna and tinned tomatoes, season with salt and pepper and stir well. Bring to the boil, then stir through the cooked pasta.

5. Tip the mixture into an ovenproof dish (approx. 23 x 15cm) or a casserole dish.

6. Top with the grated Cheddar cheese and the chopped parsley and bake for 20 minutes until bubbling. Serve.

Per serving

Carbs	of which sugars	Protein	Fat	Fibre	Kcal
64g	17g	38g	51g	12g	888kcal

Easy vegetable curry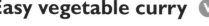

Level	Prep time	Cook time	Days in fridge	Freeze
Easy	10 minutes	30 minutes	3	Yes

Serves 2

This flexible recipe is great for using up any leftover vegetables – just add them to the pot at the right time to come together at the end. You don't need a huge list of spices and you may well have most of these ingredients in your storecupboard already. It is a great one to make in advance as it tastes even better the next day. You can eat it on its own, or serve with brown or wild rice.

3 garlic cloves, peeled
3cm fresh ginger, peeled and roughly chopped
1 onion, roughly chopped
3 tbsp coconut oil
6 sprigs fresh coriander, finely chopped, plus
    extra to garnish
pinch of salt
½ x 400g tin whole plum tomatoes
½ tsp ground turmeric
1 tsp chilli powder
1 tsp garam masala
1 x 400g tin unsweetened coconut milk
1 carrot, peeled and sliced into batons
½ cauliflower, broken into bite-size florets
1 courgette, sliced into rounds
1 handful broccoli, broken into bite-size florets
75g frozen peas
1 red chilli, sliced

1. Place the garlic, ginger and onion into a high-speed blender with 60ml water and blend to a smooth paste.

2. Melt the coconut oil in a large, heavy based saucepan over a low-medium heat. Add the paste, coriander and salt and gently fry for 5–8 minutes or until the paste starts to brown.

3. Stir in the tomatoes, turmeric and chilli powder, turn the heat to low and fry for 5 minutes more.

4. Add the garam masala and fry for a minute or two, then mix in the coconut milk and add the carrot and cauliflower. Cover the pan with a lid and then turn up the heat a little to simmer gently for 10 minutes.

5. Add the courgette and simmer for another 5 minutes.

6. Add the broccoli and the peas with 60–120ml water (depending on how you like the consistency) to loosen.

7. Simmer for 2 minutes more until the peas are cooked. Serve scattered with the sliced chilli and a few extra sprigs of coriander.

Per serving					
Carbs	of which sugars	Protein	Fat	Fibre	Kcal
39g	22g	13g	30g	13g	489kcal

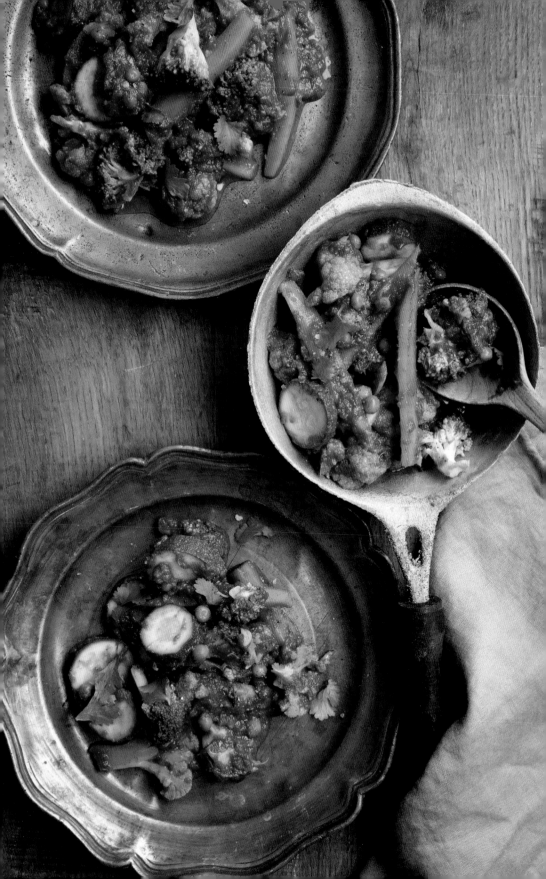

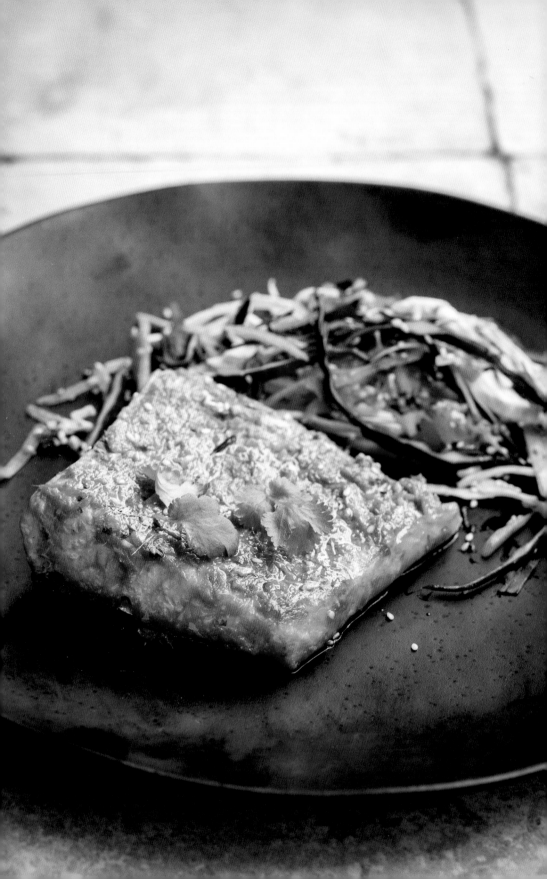

Lemongrass and ginger salmon with Asian salad

Level	Prep time	Cook time	Days in fridge	Freeze
Moderate	10 minutes	12 minutes	2	Yes

Serves 2

The combination of lemongrass and ginger gives a unique lemony, but sweet taste. They are both anti-inflammatory herbs.

2 tbsp soy sauce
1 lemongrass stalk, outer skin removed, very finely chopped
1 garlic clove, finely grated
1cm fresh ginger, peeled and grated
5 sprigs fresh coriander, stalks very finely chopped and leaves reserved for garnish
2 x 150g skinless salmon steaks or fillets

For the Asian salad
1 small carrot, peeled and grated
¼ red cabbage, finely shredded
¼ white cabbage, finely shredded
1 tsp sesame seeds
1 tsp cider vinegar
1 tsp extra virgin olive oil

1. In a small bowl, mix together the soy sauce, lemongrass, garlic, ginger and coriander stalks.

2. Place the salmon in a non-metallic dish, pour over the lemongrass and ginger mixture, cover and leave to marinate for at least 30 minutes in the fridge.

3. Preheat the oven to 180°C fan/200°C/ gas mark 6.

4. Place the salmon on a non-stick baking sheet and bake in the oven for around 12 minutes until cooked through.

5. Meanwhile, for the salad, mix together the carrot, cabbages, sesame seeds, vinegar and oil in a bowl.

6. Serve the cooked salmon alongside the Asian salad, garnished with coriander leaves.

Per serving					
Carbs	of which sugars	Protein	Fat	Fibre	Kcal
9.9g	8.8g	39g	22g	5.9g	410kcal

Homemade roasted tomato ketchup

Level	Prep time	Cook time	Days in fridge	Freeze
Easy	10 minutes	30 minutes	7	Yes

Makes approx. 500g

This is a great recipe to wean your children off shop-bought ketchups. Even the 'no added sugar and salt' versions are full of artificial sweeteners.

500g cherry tomatoes, halved or quartered
  (the reddest, ripest available)
1 red onion, cut into wedges
2 garlic cloves, unpeeled
1 tsp olive oil
1 tbsp dried oregano
1 tsp vinegar (cider or rice vinegar, etc.)
salt and freshly ground black pepper

1. Preheat the oven to 180°C fan/200°C/ gas mark 6.

2. Place the tomatoes, red onion and garlic into a large roasting tray. Pour the olive oil into your hands and massage into the tomatoes, red onion and garlic. Season well with salt and pepper.

3. Spread out well in a single layer, sprinkle with dried oregano and roast in the oven for 30 minutes until softened and slightly caramelised.

4. Transfer the roasted tomatoes and onion to a blender, discarding any liquid. Squeeze the roasted garlic out of its skin and add to the blender, discarding the skin. Blitz at full power for about 2 minutes until very smooth and thick.

5. Stir in the vinegar and adjust the seasoning to taste.

6. Cool and store in a clean glass jar in the fridge for around a week, if it lasts that long. If freezing, decant into an airtight container first.

Per serving (17g)					
Carbs	of which sugars	Protein	Fat	Fibre	Kcal
0.8g	0.7g	0g	0g	0.5g	7kcal

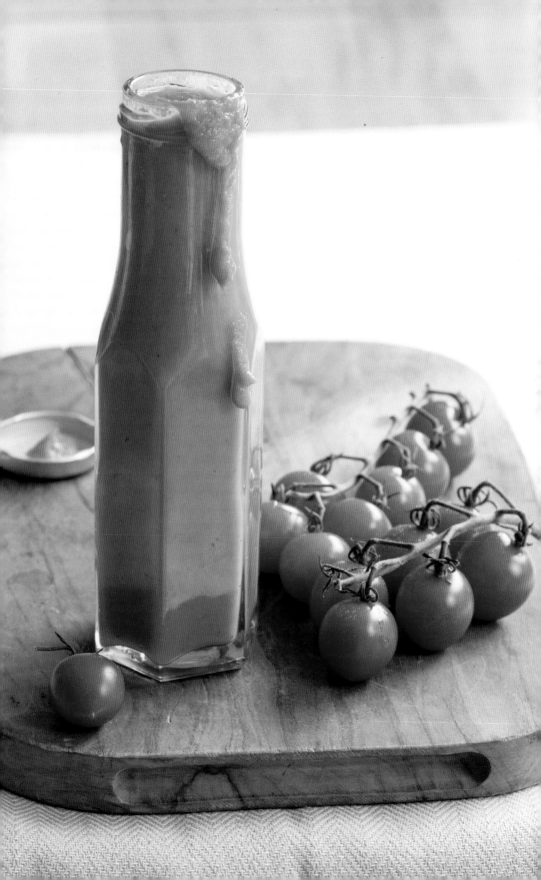

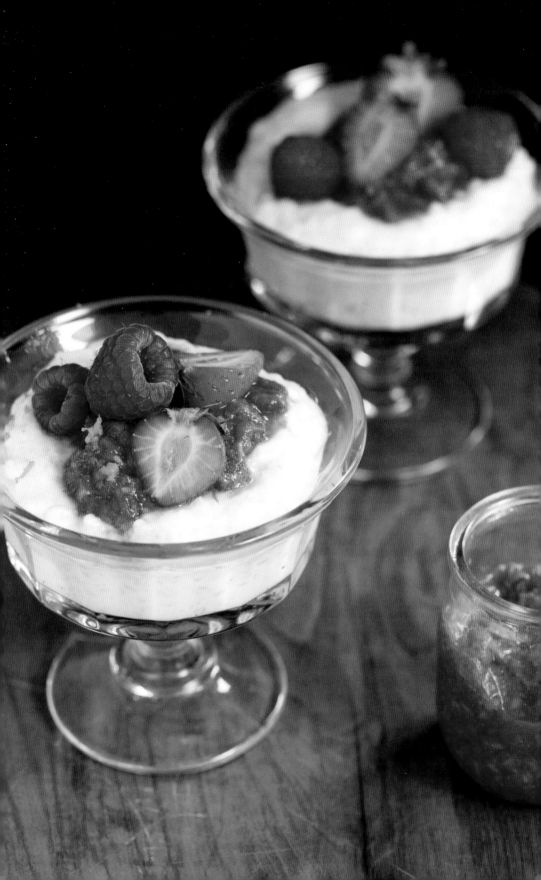

Coconut rice pudding with berry jam

Level	Prep time	Cook time	Days in fridge	Freeze
Easy	10 minutes	25 minutes	3	Yes

Serves 2

The rice pudding will keep for three days in the fridge and can be frozen for up to three months. If you want to store the jam separately, wait until it has cooled to room temperature before transferring to a clean jar. Store in the fridge for up to two weeks. The jam will thicken up and become more set once completely chilled. The jam can also be frozen for up to three months.

For the rice pudding
60g brown basmati rice
1 x 400g tin unsweetened tinned coconut milk
tiny pinch of salt
1 tsp vanilla extract

For the jam
200g fresh berries (raspberries, blueberries and/ or strawberries, etc.), plus extra to serve (optional)
grated zest and freshly squeezed juice of ½ orange, plus extra to decorate (optional)
1 tbsp ground white chia seeds

1. Place the rice into a high-speed blender and pulse a few times to break up the grains a little.

2. Place the rice in a sieve and rinse briefly.

3. Put the rice, coconut milk, a tiny pinch of salt and the vanilla into a small saucepan. Bring to the boil, then reduce the heat, cover with a lid and simmer gently for 25 minutes or until the liquid has been mostly absorbed, uncovering to stir occasionally.

4. Meanwhile, to make the jam, put the berries and orange zest and juice in a bowl and crush together with a fork. Mix in the ground chia seeds and set the jam aside to rest for 15 minutes – it will thicken as the chia seeds absorb the juices.

5. Serve the rice pudding with a dollop of the jam in each portion. Decorate with extra berries and orange zest, if you like. Keep any remaining jam in a clean glass jar in the fridge.

Per serving (based on raspberry jam and not including garnish)

Carbs	of which sugars	Protein	Fat	Fibre	Kcal
33g	7.9g	5.9g	16g	10g	326kcal

Pear and apple crumble v

Level	Prep time	Cook time	Days in fridge	Freeze
Easy	10 minutes	45 minutes	5	Yes

Serves 2

This recipe has one of the highest sugar contents in the book, which comes from the fruit. We wouldn't recommend having dessert every day, but 2–3 times per week as part of the challenge is fine if you are craving something sweet. You can also play with the sweetness using different apples, such as gala or red delicious. It also works if you throw in other fruit such as berries or rhubarb.

2 small pears, stalks and cores removed, roughly chopped into small pieces (peel or leave the skin on according to your preference)
1 eating apple, stalk and core removed, roughly chopped into small pieces (Pink Lady apples work well here)
25g unsalted butter

For the crumble topping
40g porridge oats
40g wholemeal self-raising flour
30g unsalted butter
30g pecans
25g desiccated coconut
½ tsp ground cinnamon
1 tsp vanilla extract
pinch of salt

To serve
grated zest of 1 lemon
2 heaped tbsp double cream **or** 2 heaped tbsp unsweetened Greek yoghurt

1. Preheat the oven to 180°C fan/200°C/ gas mark 6.

2. Add the pears and apple to a frying pan or saucepan with the butter and stew for about 4 minutes until the fruit is soft. It will be quicker if you have a lid for the pan.

3. Transfer the fruit to an ovenproof dish.

4. Place the topping ingredients into a food processor or mini chopper and pulse a few times to roughly chop and combine.

5. Spread the topping evenly over the fruit and then bake in the oven for 45 minutes.

6. Serve sprinkled with lemon zest and a dollop of cream or yoghurt.

Per serving (based on unpeeled fruit and double cream option 'to serve')

Carbs	of which sugars	Protein	Fat	Fibre	Kcal
51g	23g	8.4g	52g	10g	724kcal

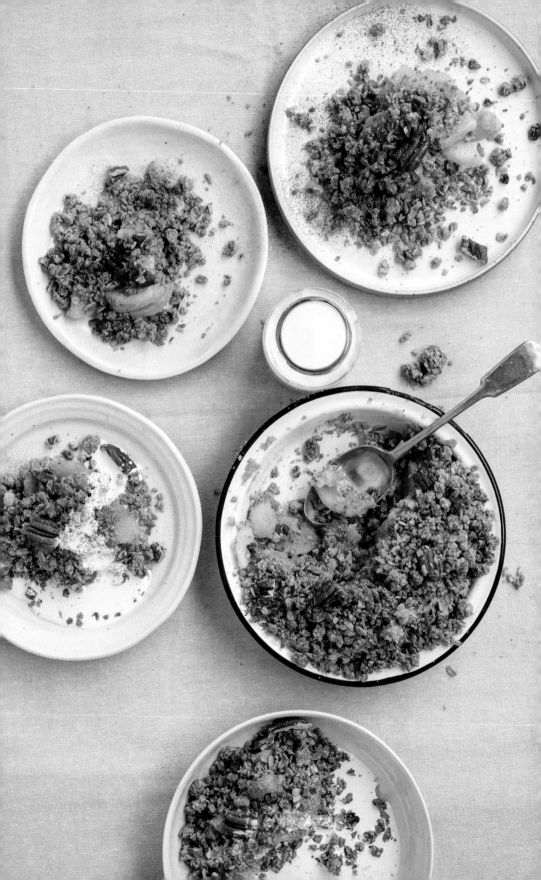

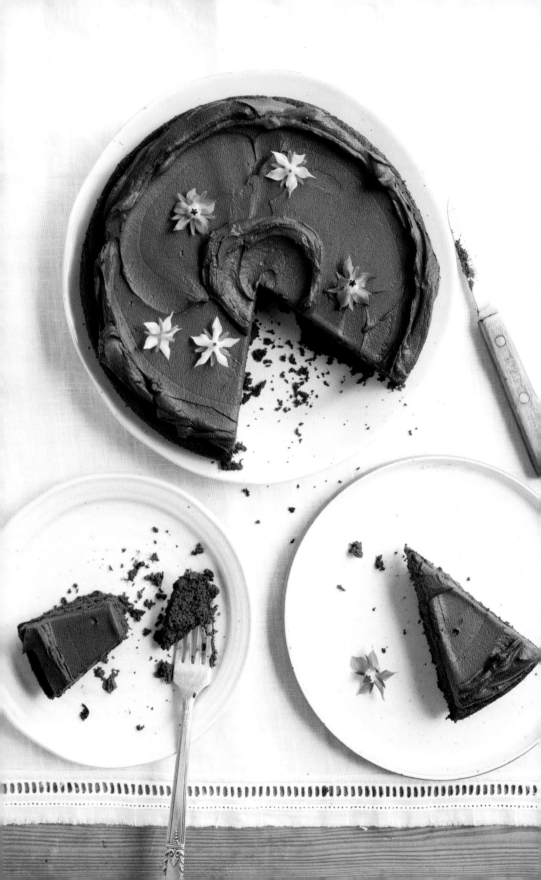

Chocolate cake v

Level	Prep time	Cook time	Days in fridge	Freeze
Moderate	10 minutes	25 minutes	5	Yes

Serves 6–8

This tastes divine! Most chocolate cake recipes are packed full of sugar, but this is a wonderful one to slowly cut the sugar content down on. You could start with a 70% cocoa solids dark chocolate bar and each time you make it slowly increase the cocoa content until you have reached 100% cocoa solids content with no added sugar. Be sure to check the sugar content on your bars as they vary wildly amongst manufacturers. You can then start to cut down on the number of dates. The optional mascarpone topping not only looks amazing, but also counteracts the slight bitterness of the dark chocolate.

100g 85% cocoa solids dark chocolate, broken into pieces
10g (1 tbsp) cacao powder
½ tsp baking powder
2 stoned dates
3 large eggs
60g unsalted butter, softened, plus extra for greasing
1 tsp vanilla extract
½ tsp salt
edible flowers, to decorate (optional)

For the topping
175g mascarpone cheese
1 tbsp cacao powder
1 tbsp full-fat milk

1. Preheat the oven to 180°C fan/200°C/gas mark 6. Grease an 18cm cake tin with butter and line the base with baking paper.

2. In a food processor, pulse the chocolate, cacao powder and baking powder together until it resembles the texture of sand.

3. Add the dates and pulse until roughly chopped and combined. If you are not using a food processor, very finely chop the chocolate and dates and combine with the cacao powder and baking powder.

4. Add the eggs, butter, vanilla extract and salt and pulse until smooth.

5. Spoon the mixture into the prepared cake tin and bake in the oven for 25 minutes until risen and a skewer inserted comes out clean.

6. Leave the cake to cool in the tin while you make the topping. Mix the mascarpone with the cacao powder and stir in the milk to loosen.

7. When the cake is completely cool, turn out of the tin and spread over the mascarpone topping with a spoon. Decorate with edible flowers, if you like.

Per serving (based on 6 servings)

Carbs	of which sugars	Protein	Fat	Fibre	Kcal
7.5g	5.2g	7.4g	34g	3.9g	370kcal

WEEK TWO

RECIPES

BREAKFASTS

Fried eggs and smashed avocado on
  sourdough
Bircher muesli
Courgette, broccoli and cheese
  scramble
Pear and chia porridge
Breakfast muffins
Giancarlo's brunch
Sweet smoothie

LUNCHES

Velvet Chinese chicken stir-fry
Baked sweet potatoes and spicy tuna
Roast cauliflower and kale salad
Minestrone soup
Pesto pasta
Crispy tofu noodle bowl

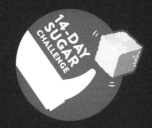

DINNERS

Fish baked in paper with creamed
 spinach
One-pot sausage casserole
Roasted Mediterranean vegetables
 and cod
Meatballs with beans and cheese
Steak and rocket
Lemon chicken
Harissa lamb burgers with courgette
 and pomegranate
Aubergine parmigiana

DESSERTS

Carrot cake
Peanut butter and banana ice cream

Fried eggs and smashed avocado on sourdough v

Level	Prep time	Cook time	Days in fridge	Freeze
Easy	5 minutes	5 minutes	0	No

Serves 2

Sourdough is a great option for your breakfast toast because it has a relatively low glycaemic index compared to other types of bread. It also contains higher levels of folate and antioxidants and less gluten than other breads. If you can find one made from whole grains, then even better.

1 large avocado, halved and stoned
1 tsp dried chilli flakes, plus extra to serve
pinch of salt
2 slices sourdough bread
1 tbsp olive oil
2 large free-range eggs
freshly ground black pepper

1. Scoop out the avocado flesh into a bowl. Add the chilli flakes, salt and some black pepper and smash together with a fork.

2. Toast the sourdough bread and top each slice with half the smashed avocado.

3. Heat the oil in a medium, non-stick frying pan and fry the eggs to your liking. Serve the fried eggs on top of the avocado toast with another twist of black pepper and extra chilli flakes to finish.

Per serving					
Carbs	of which sugars	Protein	Fat	Fibre	Kcal
16g	2.1g	11g	23g	6.2g	335kcal

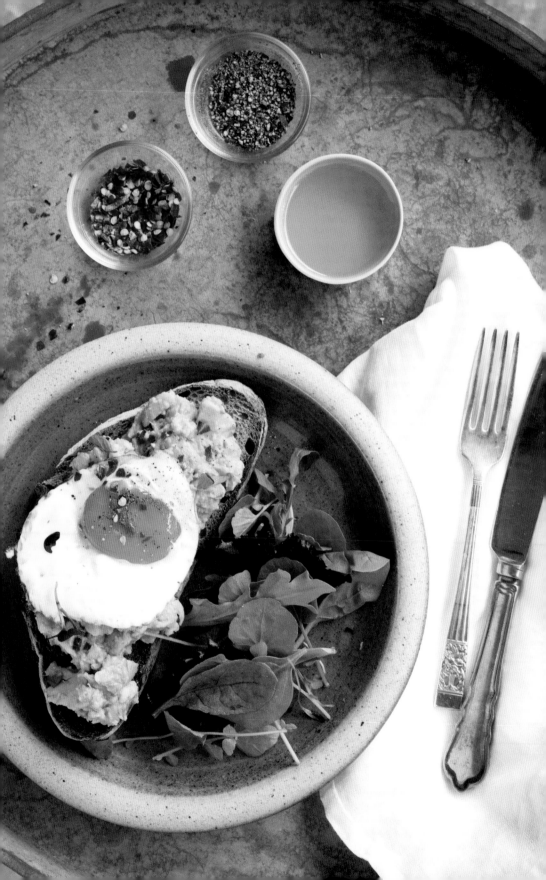

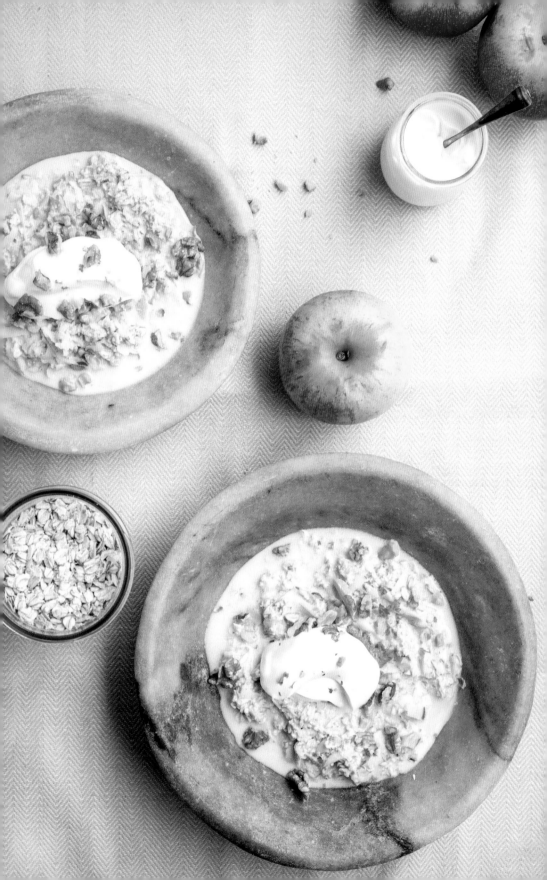

Bircher muesli v

Level	Prep time	Days in fridge	Freeze
Easy	5 minutes	5	No

Serves 2

This recipe is great because you can combine the oats, seeds and liquid the night before and refrigerate to ease the morning rush, you can even use a jam jar if you need a portable breakfast. Just add the nuts at the last minute so they keep their crunch.

50g porridge oats
30g mixed seeds (chia, sunflower, pumpkin, sesame or flaxseeds, etc.)
100ml water or unsweetened nut milk
1 Granny Smith apple, skin-on, cored and grated
4 tbsp natural Greek yoghurt (or unsweetened non-dairy yoghurt)
chopped nuts (walnuts or toasted hazelnuts, etc.), to serve

1. Soak the oats and mixed seeds in the water or nut milk for at least 15 minutes or in the fridge overnight.

2. Mix in the grated apple and yoghurt.

3. Serve sprinkled with chopped nuts.

Per serving (based on water option)

Carbs	of which sugars	Protein	Fat	Fibre	Kcal
34g	14g	21g	26g	4.6g	463kcal

Courgette, broccoli and cheese scramble v

Level	Prep time	Cook time	Days in fridge	Freeze
Easy	10 minutes	10 minutes	1	No

Serves 2

A twist on the normal scrambled eggs, full of greens! You can use up whatever cheese you have in the fridge.

2 tbsp unsalted butter
1 baby courgette, sliced into rounds
3 spring onions, sliced
1 red chilli, sliced
75g Tenderstem broccoli tips
3 large free-range eggs, lightly beaten
75g mixed grated or shaved cheese (Cheddar, mozzarella, Gruyère, Parmesan, etc.)
small handful of green herbs leaves (parsley, coriander or basil, etc.)
salt and freshly ground black pepper

1. Melt the butter in a large, non-stick frying pan over a medium heat. Once the butter is foaming, add the courgette slices in one layer and cook for a few minutes until golden underneath. Turn them, then mix in the spring onions, chilli and broccoli and season with salt and black pepper. Fry for 2–3 minutes to slightly soften the vegetables.

2. Add the eggs and cheese and stir through, cooking for another 2–3 minutes until the eggs are just set.

3. Scatter the scramble with the green herb leaves and serve.

Per serving (based on Cheddar option)					
Carbs	of which sugars	Protein	Fat	Fibre	Kcal
5g	3.5g	25g	34g	5.7g	439kcal

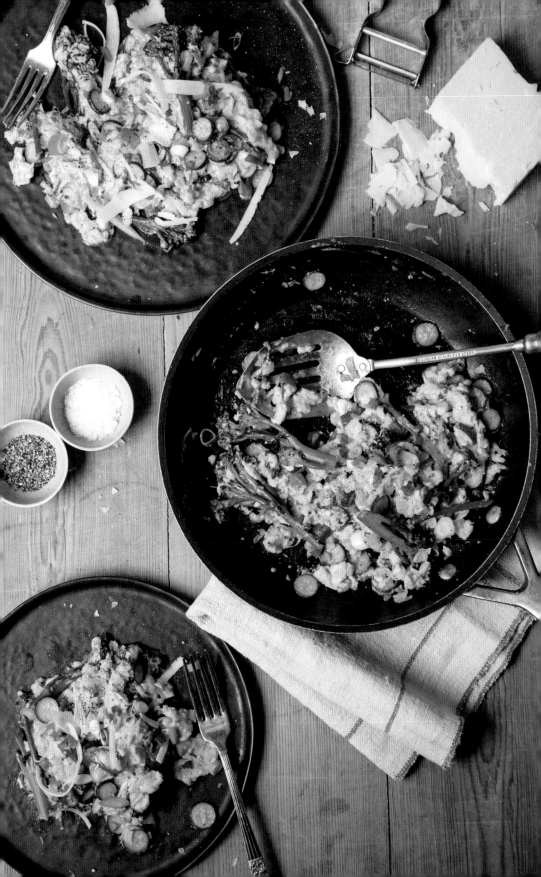

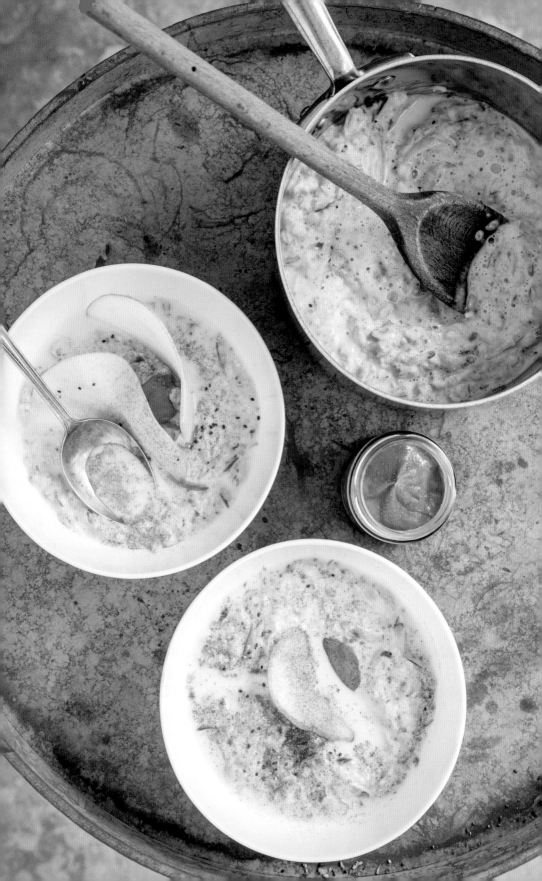

Pear and chia porridge Ⓥ

Level	Prep time	Cook time	Days in fridge	Freeze
Easy	5 minutes	10 minutes	3	No

Serves 2

There are many varieties of porridge oats, including rolled, quick and instant. Regardless of the type, all porridge oats are whole grains, which provide you with slow-releasing energy throughout the morning. The cooking time will depend on which oats you choose, so please check instructions on the packet.

You can make this recipe dairy-free with water rather than milk, if you prefer; this would also reduce the fat, protein and calorie content.

80g rolled porridge oats
1 tbsp chia seeds
2 pears, skin on, cored and grated, reserving a little grated or sliced to decorate
400ml dairy milk or nut milk
1¼ tsp ground cinnamon
tiny pinch of salt
2 tbsp unsweetened nut butter (cashew, almond or peanut, etc.), to serve

1. Place the oats, chia seeds, pears, milk, cinnamon and salt into a small saucepan over a low heat and bring to a gentle simmer. Cook for 3–4 minutes, stirring continuously, until creamy and thickened.

2. Serve each portion topped with a swirl of your favourite nut butter, and a little reserved grated or sliced pear, if you like.

Per serving (based on peanut butter and semi-skimmed milk options)

Carbs	of which sugars	Protein	Fat	Fibre	Kcal
51g	22g	17g	21g	9.5g	477kcal

Breakfast muffins v

Level	Prep time	Cook time	Days in storage	Freeze
Moderate	10 minutes	25 minutes	3	Yes

Makes 6 large muffins

If you cannot find wholemeal self-raising flour, you can use plain wholemeal flour and add 1½ tsp baking powder. We used Granny Smiths but any eating apple will work. You could also add 2 tbsp mixed seed (such as pumpkin, sunflower and flaxseed) or walnuts into the mixture to give it extra nutrients and more bite.

150g unsalted butter
2 eating apples, peeled, cored and grated
2 bananas, peeled and mashed
300g wholemeal self-raising flour
2 free-range eggs, lightly beaten
2 tsp baking powder
1½ tsp ground cinnamon

1. Preheat the oven to 160°C fan/180°C/ gas mark 4 and line a 6-hole muffin tray with paper cases.

2. Melt the butter in a small saucepan over a medium heat. Add the grated apples and cook for 5 minutes until softened.

3. Tip into a mixing bowl with the remaining ingredients and mix well.

4. Spoon the mixture into the paper cases, dividing it evenly, and then bake in the oven for 20 minutes until risen and pale golden. Leave to cool before serving.

Per muffin (based on making 6 muffins)

Carbs	of which sugars	Protein	Fat	Fibre	Kcal
44g	11g	9g	23g	1.5g	426kcal

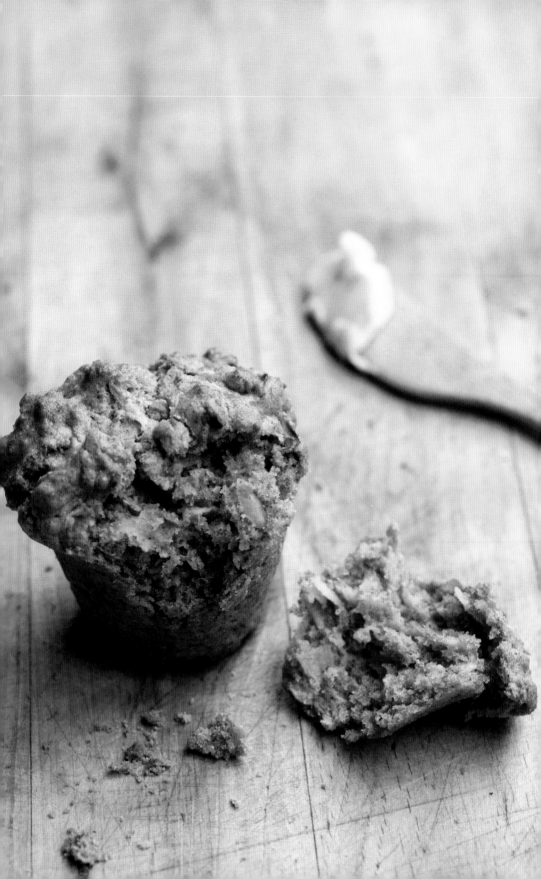

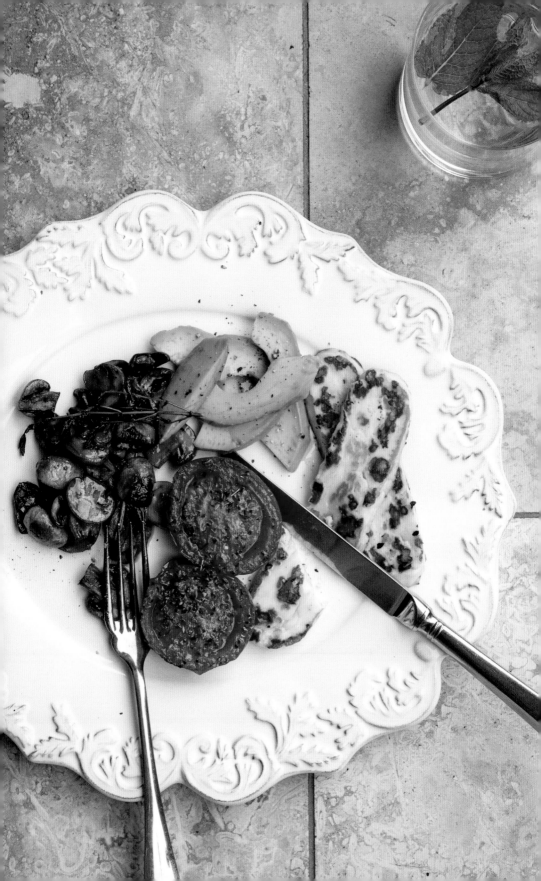

Giancarlo's brunch v

Level	Prep time	Cook time	Days in fridge	Freeze
Moderate	15 minutes	20 minutes	0	No

Serves 4

This recipe has been kindly donated by Giancarlo Caldesi from his book *The Diabetes Weight-loss Cookbook*. The herbs bring loads of flavour to the mushrooms and it is a great weekend treat.

400g fresh tomatoes, halved
2 tbsp olive oil
pinch of dried oregano
2 garlic cloves, finely chopped
3 sprigs fresh thyme
3 sprigs fresh rosemary
1 red chilli, finely chopped
500g chestnut mushrooms, chopped
225g halloumi, cut into 1cm-thick slices
1 avocado, peeled, stoned and sliced
salt and freshly ground black pepper

1. Preheat the oven to 180°C fan/200°C/gas mark 6.

2. Toss the tomatoes with ½ tbsp of the olive oil and the oregano and season with salt and black pepper. Spread evenly in a baking tray and bake for 15–20 minutes until softened.

3. Meanwhile, heat the remaining 1½ tbsp oil in a large frying pan over a high heat. Add the garlic, thyme, rosemary and chilli and season with salt and black pepper. Fry for 1 minute, then add the mushrooms and cook over a high heat, stirring frequently, for 10 minutes or until most of the juices have evaporated. Keep warm until needed.

4. Place a separate non-stick frying pan over a medium-high heat. Add the halloumi slices to the pan and dry-fry for a couple of minutes, then turn over and cook for another 2 minutes until brown on both sides.

5. Serve the halloumi with the roasted tomatoes, fried mushrooms and sliced avocado.

Per serving					
Carbs	of which sugars	Protein	Fat	Fibre	Kcal
11g	6.5g	18g	27g	3.5g	364kcal

Sweet smoothie v

Level	Prep time	Days in fridge	Freeze
Easy	5 minutes	1	Yes

Serves 2

This is a great way of giving you a morning vitamin boost, and with the oats, can be breakfast on the go. You can use frozen strawberries if you are making this out of season. This contains more vegetables to ensure it has low acidity to protect your teeth. Always rinse for 20 seconds with water after having acidic smoothies.

5 strawberries, stalks removed, plus extra sliced to decorate (optional)
200g leafy green vegetables (spinach, watercress, chard or rocket, etc.), plus extra to decorate (optional)
50g Greek yoghurt (or unsweetened non-dairy yoghurt)
20g rolled oats
1 tbsp chia seeds, plus extra to decorate (optional)

1. Place all of the ingredients into a blender and blitz until smooth. Pour into glasses to serve. Decorate with extra sliced strawberry, spinach and a tiny sprinkling of chia seeds, if you like.

Per serving (based on Greek yoghurt option without the garnish)

Carbs	of which sugars	Protein	Fat	Fibre	Kcal
10g	3g	7.5g	3.2g	5g	110kcal

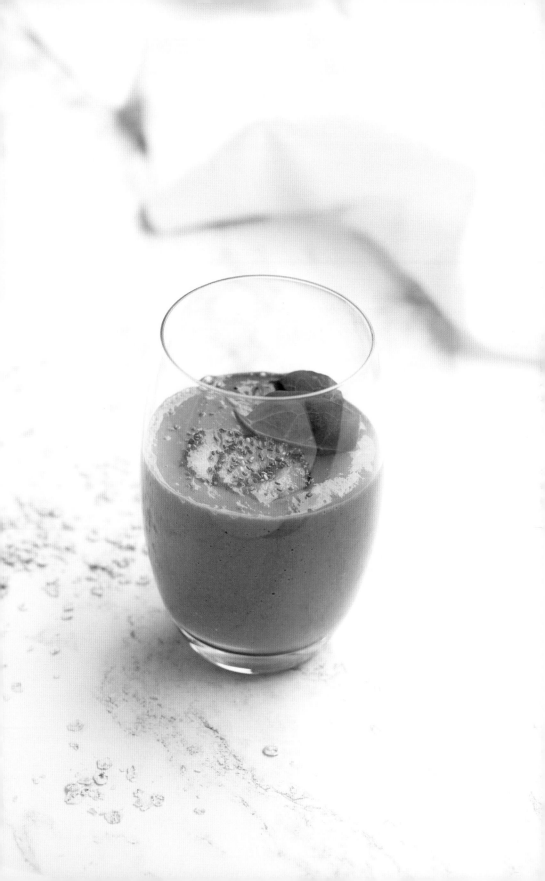

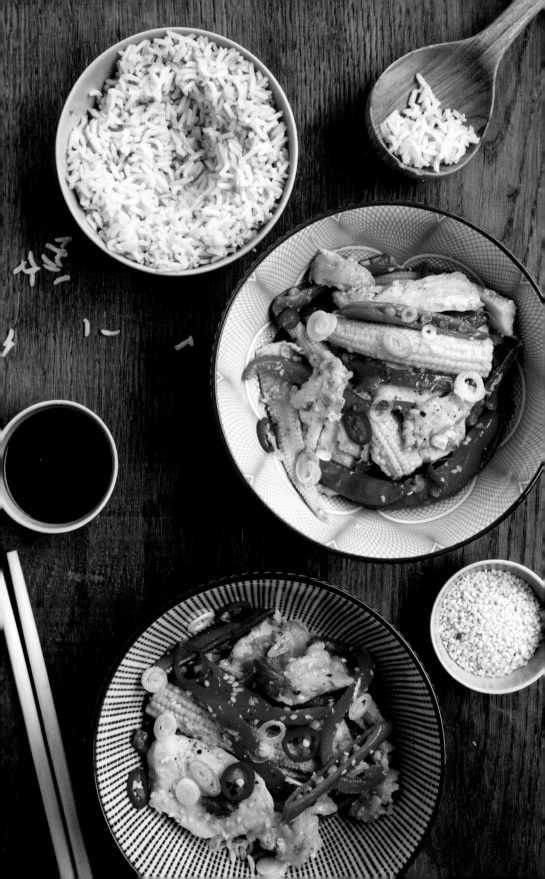

Velvet Chinese chicken stir-fry

Level	Prep time	Cook time	Days in fridge	Freeze
Moderate	15 minutes	30–40 minutes	1	No

Serves 2

'Velveting' comes from Chinese cooking, it is a type of marinade that makes meat or seafood so much softer with a silky texture. It is well worth the extra ten minutes of preparation. You could also serve this with our yummy cauliflower rice.

2 free-range eggs
2 tsp cornflour
2 chicken breasts, cut into bite-size pieces
150g brown basmati rice
1 tbsp sesame oil
3 tbsp groundnut or coconut oil
4 spring onions, finely sliced
2 garlic cloves, finely grated
2 tbsp soy sauce, plus extra to serve
1 red pepper, deseeded and cut into thin strips
100g baby corn, each sliced into 4 lengthways
75g sugar snap peas, sliced diagonally
salt and freshly ground black pepper
sliced red chilli, to serve (optional)

1. To velvet the chicken, separate the white from one of the eggs (save the yolk) and mix together in a bowl with the cornflour and a pinch of salt. Mix in the chicken, cover and refrigerate for 10 minutes.

2. Rinse the rice in a sieve under cold water until the water runs clear. This helps remove loose starch so the rice will be less sticky. Place in a medium-sized saucepan. Add 500ml water and a generous pinch of salt. Put over a high heat and bring to a rapid boil. Stir the rice, then cover the pan with a tight-fitting lid and reduce the heat to a low simmer. Cook for 30–40 minutes (or according to the packet instructions) until the water has been absorbed and the rice is cooked.

3. Meanwhile, place the remaining egg yolk and whole egg into another bowl, season with salt and black pepper and ½ tbsp of the sesame oil, beat lightly and set aside.

4. Put the groundnut or coconut oil in a large, heavy-based frying pan over a medium heat. Add the chicken pieces (discarding any excess marinade). Turn the chicken after about 3 minutes once it releases from the pan. Cook on the other side for a minute or two.

5. Increase the heat and add the spring onions and garlic, then stir in the soy sauce with 2–3 tbsp water. Add the red pepper, baby corn and sugar snap peas and stir-fry for a minute or two.

6. Push everything to one side of the pan, add the seasoned egg in the space and let it fry without stirring until set like an omelette, then break it up with the spoon and mix through the rest of the ingredients. Finish the stir-fry with the remaining sesame oil and extra soy sauce, if liked. Serve immediately with black pepper and the cooked brown basmati rice. Top with sliced red chilli, if you like.

Per serving

Carbs	of which sugars	Protein	Fat	Fibre	Kcal
62g	6.6g	49g	54g	7.3g	941kcal

Baked sweet potatoes and spicy tuna

Level	Prep time	Cook time	Days in fridge	Freeze
Easy	10 minutes	30–40 minutes	2	No

Serves 2

This is a spin on the normal white baked potato. Whilst they both have similar carbohydrate content, the sweet potato has more fibre and micronutrients and is lower on the glycaemic index than white potatoes. Your blood glucose levels will rise a little more gradually with sweet potatoes than with white potatoes.

2 sweet potatoes, skins scrubbed and dried
1 x 200g tin tuna in olive oil
1 small red onion, very finely chopped
1 red chilli, finely chopped
handful fresh coriander, finely chopped
2 heaped tbsp natural Greek yoghurt
   (or unsweetened non-dairy yoghurt)
salt and freshly ground black pepper
mixed salad leaves, to serve

1. Preheat the oven to 190°C fan/210°C/ gas mark 6.

2. Place the sweet potatoes into the oven directly on the shelf and bake for 30–40 minutes until soft all the way through.

3. Meanwhile, put the tuna and its oil, the red onion, chilli and coriander in a bowl and mix.

4. Season the yoghurt with salt and black pepper in a separate bowl.

5. Put the baked sweet potatoes on serving plates, slice open and top with the spicy tuna and a dollop of seasoned yoghurt. Serve with mixed salad leaves on the side.

Per serving (without salad leaves)

Carbs	of which sugars	Protein	Fat	Fibre	Kcal
32g	19g	32g	6.9g	3.6g	328kcal

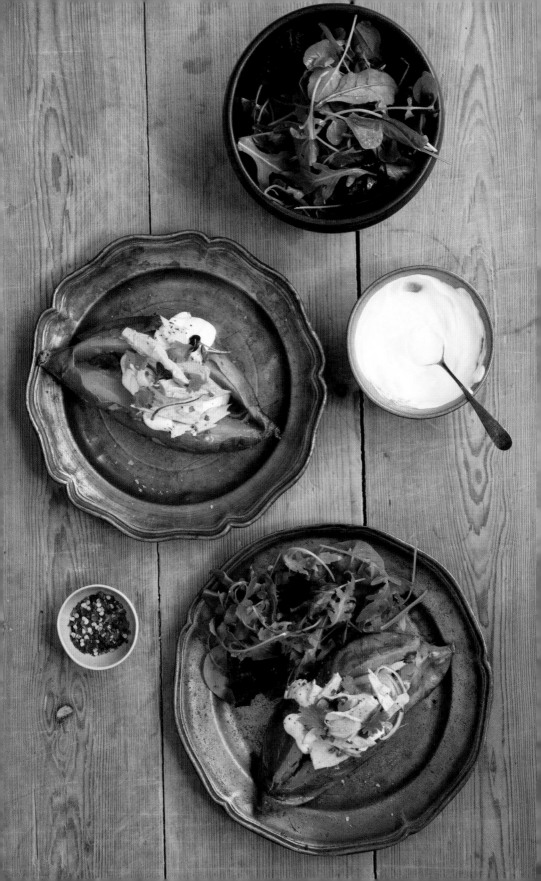

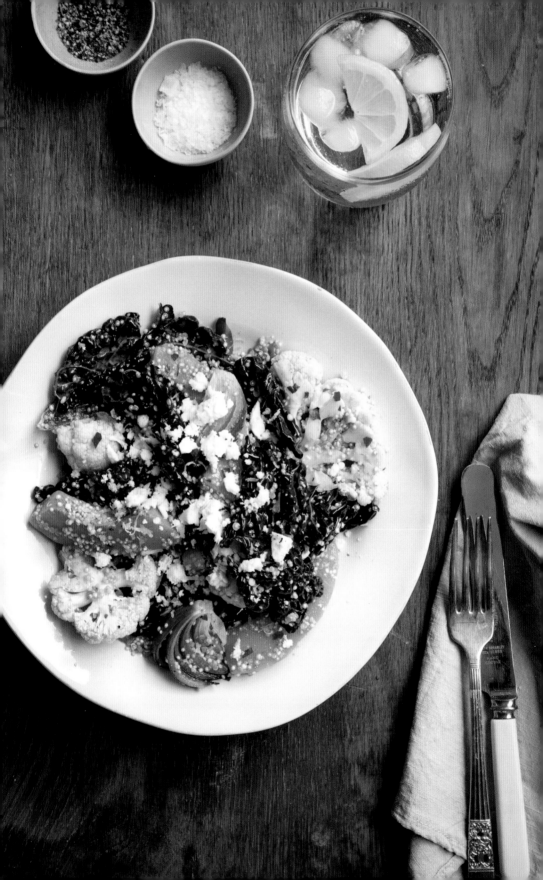

Roast cauliflower and kale salad v

Level	Prep time	Cook time	Days in fridge	Freeze
Easy	10 minutes	30 minutes	3	No

Serves 2

Kale is a type of cabbage that comes in two forms: kale, which has smooth leaves, and curly kale, which has crinkly leaves. You can use either in this salad but please discard the tough stalks.

½ cauliflower, florets cut into 1cm-thick slices
¼ butternut squash, peeled, deseeded and cut into thick semi-circles (approx. 200g prepared weight)
1 red onion, sliced into semi-circles
3 tbsp olive oil
1 tsp ground cumin
1 tsp dried chilli flakes
75g raw quinoa, rinsed thoroughly
100g kale, chopped
grated zest and freshly squeezed juice of ½ lemon
70g feta cheese, crumbled
salt and freshly ground black pepper

1. Preheat the oven to 180°C fan/200°C/gas mark 6.

2. Put the cauliflower, butternut squash and red onion into a large baking tray. Add 1½ tbsp of the olive oil, the cumin, dried chilli flakes and some salt and black pepper and toss together (using your hands makes this easier). Roast in the oven for 30 minutes until the vegetables are tender with a nice brown colour.

3. Meanwhile, place the quinoa into a large saucepan with 200ml water and bring to the boil. Reduce the heat to the lowest setting and half-cover the pan with a lid. Simmer gently for about 10–12 minutes until the water has been absorbed and the quinoa is cooked. Switch off the heat and stir the kale into the pan, then cover and leave for 5–8 minutes to soften.

4. Place the roasted vegetables and quinoa and kale mixture into a large bowl and drizzle with the remaining oil. Add the lemon zest and juice and mix well.

5. Pile onto plates and serve warm, topped with crumbled feta and extra black pepper.

Per serving					
Carbs	of which sugars	Protein	Fat	Fibre	Kcal
42g	17g	18g	31g	12g	544kcal

Minestrone soup v

Level	Prep time	Cook time	Days in fridge	Freeze
Easy	10 minutes	35 minutes	5	Yes

Serves 2

A very hearty soup. We used stelline or little stars pasta but you could use any shaped pasta that you have in your cupboard. To reduce the carb content you could always leave the pasta out. Or to add extra saltiness you could finish with some grated cheese.

2 tbsp olive oil
1 red onion, finely chopped
2 carrots, peeled and chopped
2 celery stalks, sliced
2 garlic cloves, finely chopped
1 bay leaf
1 courgette, sliced into semi-circles
1 x 400g tin cannellini beans, drained
1 x 400g tin whole plum tomatoes
1 litre hot vegetable stock
100g small dried wholewheat pasta
1 sprig basil, leaves picked
salt and freshly ground black pepper

1. Put the olive oil in a large soup pot over a medium-high heat. Add the red onion, carrots and celery and a pinch each of salt and black pepper and sauté for 5–6 minutes until the vegetables are soft.

2. Reduce the heat to low, then add the garlic, bay leaf, courgette, beans and tomatoes and simmer gently for 10 minutes, stirring frequently.

3. Pour in the hot vegetable stock and add the pasta. Bring to the boil and then reduce the heat and simmer for a further 15 minutes, or until the pasta is al dente, before serving scattered with fresh basil leaves.

Per serving					
Carbs	of which sugars	Protein	Fat	Fibre	Kcal
40g	12g	12g	8.7g	11g	308kcal

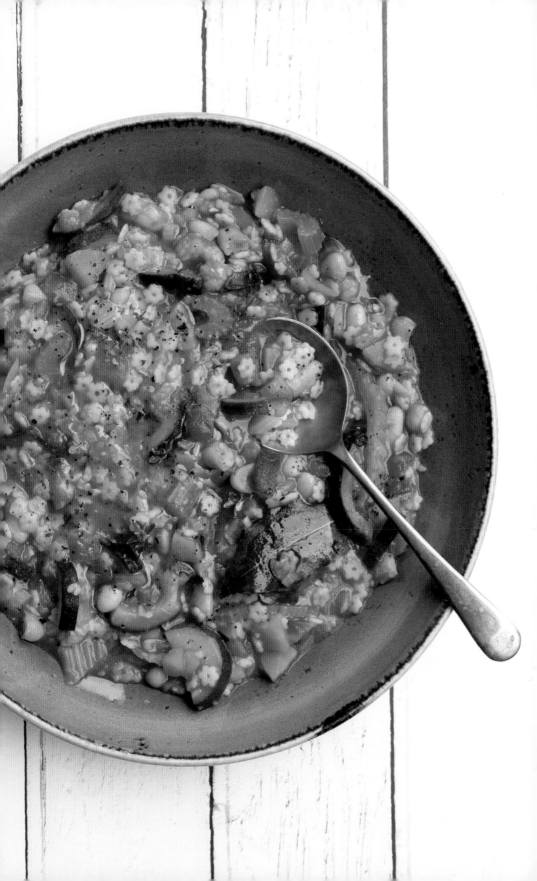

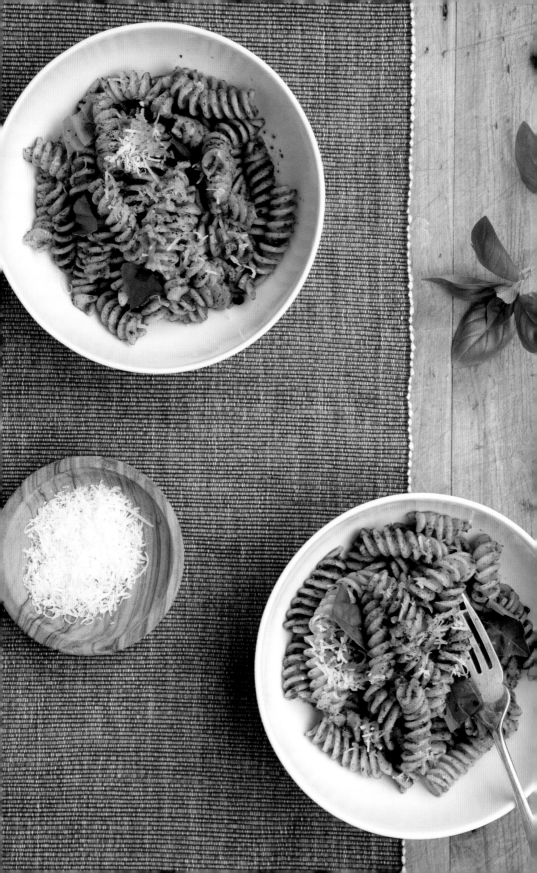

Pesto pasta

Level	Prep time	Cook time	Days in fridge	Freeze
Moderate	10 minutes	10 minutes	7	Yes

Serves 2

This pesto recipe will make more than you need for two servings, so put the remaining pesto into a clean jar, top up with a little olive oil to completely cover, and refrigerate.

200g wholewheat dried pasta (fusilli, penne, farfalle, etc.)
50g fresh basil leaves, plus extra to garnish
1 garlic clove, peeled
50g pine nuts
125ml extra virgin olive oil
25g Parmesan cheese, grated
salt and freshly ground black pepper

1. Bring a large saucepan of water to the boil, then add a pinch of salt and the pasta. Cook for about 10 minutes or according to the packet instructions. Drain the pasta and return to the pan.

2. Meanwhile, put the basil, garlic and pine nuts into a food processor or mini chopper and blitz to a paste. Stir in the extra virgin olive oil, followed by the Parmesan. Season with salt and black pepper to taste.

3. Stir a few spoonfuls of pesto into the hot drained pasta and serve with plenty of extra black pepper. Garnish with basil leaves.

Per serving					
Carbs	of which sugars	Protein	Fat	Fibre	Kcal
64g	4.7g	23g	87g	10g	1145kcal

Crispy tofu noodle bowl

Level	Prep time	Cook time	Days in fridge	Freeze
Moderate	15 minutes	15 minutes	2	No

Serves 2

Despite the name, buckwheat noodles are wheat- and gluten-free and taste delicious.

For the dressing
1 garlic clove, finely grated
thumb-sized piece fresh ginger, peeled and grated
2 tbsp olive oil
1 tbsp soy sauce
1 large red chilli, sliced

For the noodle bowl
200g good-quality firm tofu, drained
2 tsp cornflour
2 tsp sesame oil
1 courgette, sliced into ribbons with a peeler or mandoline
1 orange or purple carrot, peeled and sliced into ribbons with a peeler or mandoline
6 sprigs fresh coriander, roughly torn
100g dried soba (100% buckwheat) noodles
grated zest and freshly squeezed juice of 1 lime

1. Put all the dressing ingredients into a clean jam jar and shake to combine. If you don't have a jam jar, then simply whisk them together in a small bowl. Set aside.

2. Preheat the oven to 180°C fan/200°C/gas mark 6.

3. Squeeze out the excess water from the tofu into kitchen paper. Chop the tofu into bite-size chunks, then roll the chunks in the cornflour to evenly coat all over.

4. Place 1 tsp of the sesame oil in a frying pan over a medium-high heat. Add the tofu and fry, turning occasionally, until crisp and golden on all sides. Remove to a plate covered with kitchen paper to drain off the excess oil.

5. Place the courgette, carrot and coriander onto a baking tray and drizzle with the remaining 1 tsp sesame oil. Bake in the oven for 2–3 minutes until very slightly softened.

6. Meanwhile, bring a large saucepan of water to the boil and add the noodles. Lower the heat and simmer gently for 5 minutes, no longer. Drain and rinse the noodles under cold water.

7. Place the noodles, vegetables and fried tofu in a large bowl. Add the lime zest and squeeze over the lime juice and then drizzle over the dressing. Toss together.

8. Serve immediately in two bowls with chopsticks, if you like.

Per serving					
Carbs	of which sugars	Protein	Fat	Fibre	Kcal
45g	4.9g	19g	20g	8.2g	458kcal

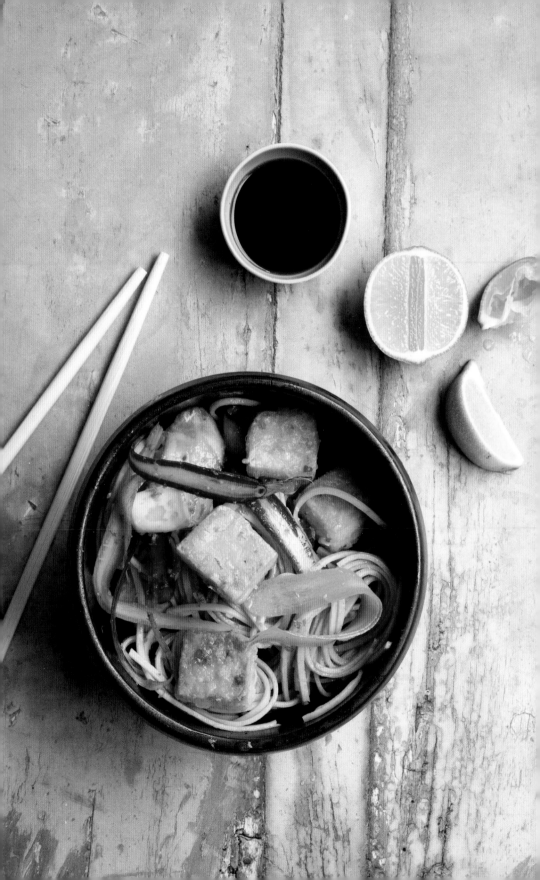

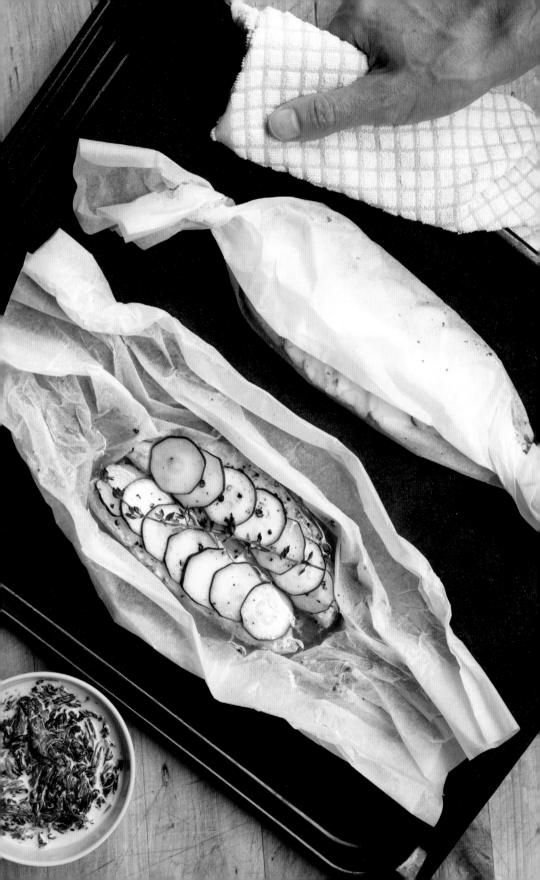

Fish baked in paper with creamed spinach

Level	Prep time	Cook time	Days in fridge	Freeze
Moderate	10 minutes	10 minutes	1	No

Serves 2

Cooking fish in paper in the oven in its own juices is so delicious, simple and quick. It makes minimal mess, so the clean up operation afterwards is also quick.

2 fresh mackerel or salmon fillets, skin on
1 tbsp olive oil
1 courgette, sliced into very thin rounds
2 thyme sprigs
salt and freshly ground black pepper

For the creamed spinach
1 tbsp unsalted butter
200g spinach
75ml double cream
3 tbsp grated Parmesan cheese
a little freshly grated nutmeg or ¼ tsp
    ground nutmeg

1. Preheat the oven to 200°C fan/220°C/gas mark 7.

2. Smear the fish skin with the olive oil using a pastry brush or a spoon and season with salt and pepper. Put each fish fillet on a separate piece of baking paper, skin-side down, then place on a baking tray. Add the slices of courgette on top of each fish fillet, slightly overlapping one another and top with a sprig of thyme.

3. Fold over the paper and twist the edges like a cracker to make two fish parcels. Bake the fish in the oven for about 10 minutes or until it is cooked through.

4. Meanwhile, for the creamed spinach, melt the butter in a large frying pan over a medium heat. Tip in the spinach and let it wilt for about 5 minutes until all the water has evaporated. Stir in the double cream and Parmesan. Season with salt and black pepper and add a little nutmeg.

5. Put the creamed spinach onto serving plates and sit the cooked fish on top to serve.

Per serving					
Carbs	of which sugars	Protein	Fat	Fibre	Kcal
3.1g	2.6g	28g	50g	3.2g	583kcal

One-pot sausage casserole

Level	Prep time	Cook time	Days in fridge	Freeze
Easy	5 minutes	15–17 minutes	3	Yes

Serves 2

This super speedy mid-week dish is perfect for when you are in a hurry to get food on the table. For a meat-free option, just use good-quality vegetarian sausages.

2 tbsp olive oil
2 red onions, cut into wedges
1 garlic clove, finely chopped
12 good-quality chipolatas (at least 90% meat content)
1 x 400g tin borlotti beans, drained
200g Speedy Tomato Sauce (see page 95)
few sprigs fresh parsley, leaves only, chopped

1. Put the oil in a large frying pan or casserole dish over a medium heat. Add the onions and fry for 5 minutes until softened. Add the garlic and fry for 1 minute more.

2. Add the sausages whole and fry for 5 minutes more until they are golden brown.

3. Add the beans and tomato sauce and bring to the boil, then lower the heat and simmer for 5–6 minutes.

4. Scatter with the parsley and serve.

Per serving					
Carbs	of which sugars	Protein	Fat	Fibre	Kcal
45g	12g	42g	50g	17g	837kcal

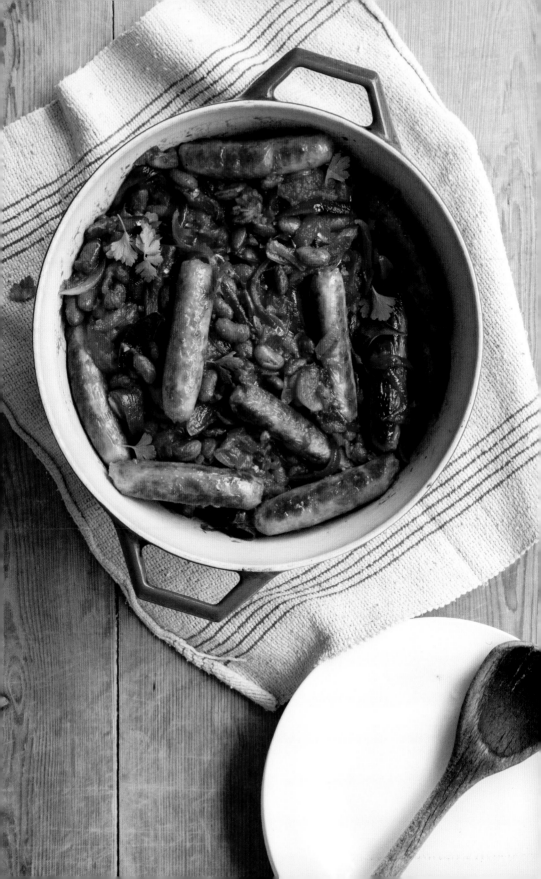

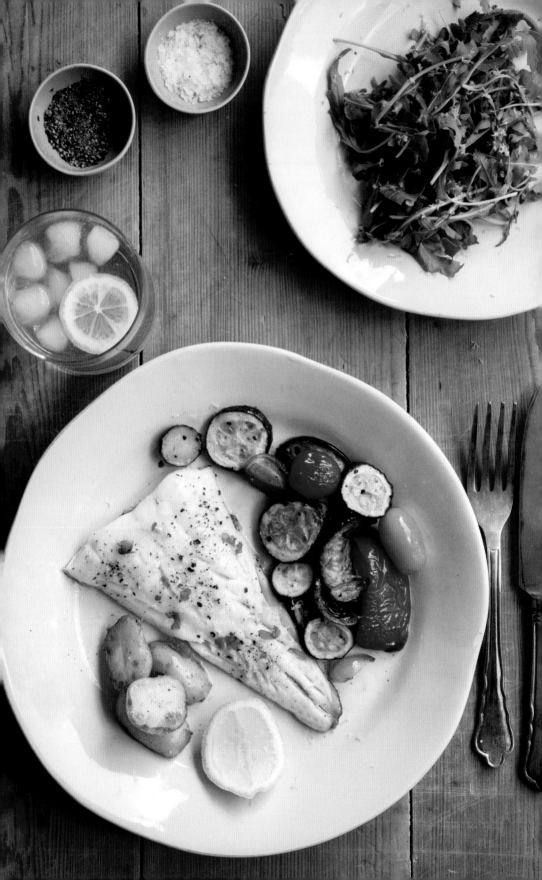

Roasted Mediterranean vegetables and cod

Level	Prep time	Cook time	Days in fridge	Freeze
Moderate	10 minutes	30–40 minutes	2	No

Serves 2

If you have the time, it is a great idea to make a double batch of these roasted vegetables, which you can eat cold for lunch the next day topped with feta.

250g baby new potatoes, halved
1 red onion, cut into wedges
1 red pepper, deseeded and cut into chunks
200g cherry tomatoes
1 aubergine, cut into chunks
1 courgette, sliced
3 tbsp olive oil, plus an extra drizzle for the fish
2 x 125g cod fillets
2 slices of lemon
salt and freshly ground black pepper

1. Blanch the baby potatoes in a large saucepan of boiling water for about 3–5 minutes until softened, then drain.

2. Preheat the oven to 200°C fan/220°C/gas mark 7.

3. Place all of the vegetables with the potatoes into a large bowl. Add the oil and some salt and black pepper and toss together.

4. Tip onto one or two baking trays in one flat layer so they are not too crowded. Roast in the oven for 30–40 minutes until the potatoes are crisp and the veg are slightly caramelised.

5. Meanwhile, top each piece of cod with a slice of lemon, season with salt and black pepper and add a drizzle of oil. Place on baking paper on another baking tray and add the fish to the oven for the last 12 minutes of the vegetable cooking time to roast.

6. Serve the cod with the roasted vegetables.

Per serving					
Carbs	of which sugars	Protein	Fat	Fibre	Kcal
34g	16g	30g	21g	11g	474kcal

Meatballs with beans and cheese

Level	Prep time	Cook time	Days in fridge	Freeze
Moderate	15 minutes	35–45 minutes	3	Yes

Serves 2

To keep meatballs from falling apart it's best to work with a well-chilled mixture, to work quickly and handle them as little as possible so they don't warm up. You can mix together all the ingredients, roll into balls and chill them for at least 15 minutes and up to an hour before baking in the oven.

400g minced beef and/or pork
½ onion, finely grated
15g Parmesan cheese, grated, plus extra to serve (optional)
1 small free-range egg, lightly beaten
1 tbsp olive oil
300g Speedy Tomato Sauce (see page 95)
1 x 400g tin beans, drained (black beans, adzuki beans or haricot beans, etc.)
70g cheese, grated (mozzarella or Cheddar, etc.)
salt and freshly ground black pepper

To serve
1 tsp freshly chopped parsley
1 tsp freshly chopped basil
1 tsp dried oregano
50g baby spinach leaves

1. Place the minced meat into a bowl with the onion, Parmesan, egg, ½ tbsp of the oil and some salt and black pepper. Mix together very thoroughly using your hands. Take small handfuls of the mixture (approx. 40g each) and roll firmly into about 12–15 meatballs.

2. Preheat the oven to 180°C fan/200°C/gas mark 6.

3. Place the remaining ½ tbsp oil at the bottom of an ovenproof dish and toss the meatballs in it to coat in oil. Season again and then refrigerate the meatballs in the dish until ready to cook, ideally at least 15 minutes.

4. Bake the meatballs in their dish for 20–30 minutes until they have some colour, shaking the dish halfway through.

5. Remove from the oven and stir in the tomato sauce, beans and 50ml water. Top with the grated cheese and return to the oven for 15 minutes or until bubbling.

6. Sprinkle with the parsley, basil and oregano and extra grated Parmesan, if you like. Serve alongside the baby spinach leaves.

Per serving (not including extra Parmesan cheese)

Carbs	of which sugars	Protein	Fat	Fibre	Kcal
33g	16g	77g	38g	21g	832kcal

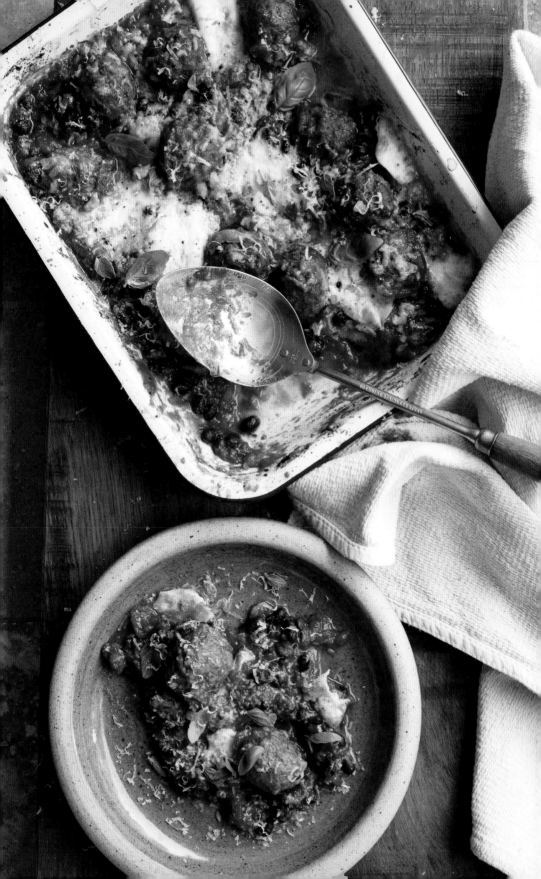

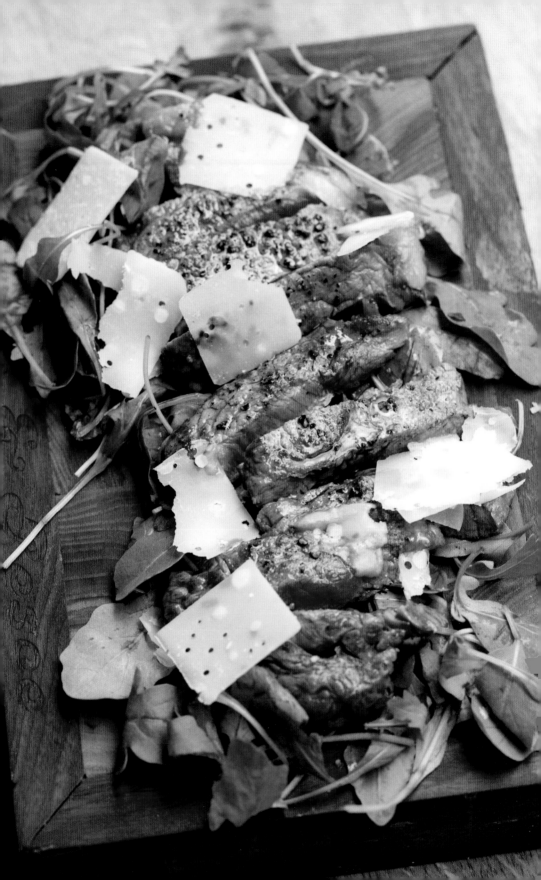

Steak and rocket

Level	Prep time	Cook time	Days in fridge	Freeze
Easy	5 minutes	5–10 minutes	3	No

Serves 1

This recipe is from the cookbook *Return to Tuscany*. It came about after the documentary series following Giancarlo and Katie Caldesi as they strived to make a success of a cookery school in Tuscany. We were one of the first guests at the school, where we learnt to make this simple dish.

1 x 250g sirloin steak
2 tbsp olive oil
40g mixed salad leaves
50g cherry tomatoes, sliced (optional)
2 tbsp good-quality balsamic vinegar
20g Parmesan cheese, shaved with a peeler or cut into thin slices
salt and freshly ground black pepper

1. Sprinkle the steak with a little salt. Heat the olive oil in a large griddle or frying pan over a high heat until very hot. Cook the steak for 2–4 minutes on each side, depending on how you like it, then remove from the pan and rest for a few minutes.

2. Arrange the salad leaves on a plate, along with the cherry tomatoes, if using.

3. Cut the steak into 2cm-thick slices and arrange over the salad. Drizzle over the balsamic vinegar and scatter with the Parmesan. Serve immediately, seasoned with black pepper.

Per serving					
Carbs	of which sugars	Protein	Fat	Fibre	Kcal
2.9g	2.7g	34g	21g	0.7g	344kcal

Lemon chicken

Level	Prep time	Cook time	Days in fridge	Freeze
Easy	10 minutes	25 minutes	3	Yes

Serves 2

We like to use chicken thighs with the skin on for this recipe to get tender and juicy chicken full of flavour. You can serve this with a salad, roasted vegetables or steamed green beans. If you cannot find buckwheat flour you could use spelt flour instead.

4 free-range skin-on bone-in chicken thighs
2 tbsp buckwheat flour
1 tbsp olive oil
2 garlic cloves, peeled
1 red chilli, finely chopped
2 small sprigs fresh thyme
100ml white wine
grated zest and freshly squeezed juice of
  1 lemon
salt and freshly ground black pepper

1. Season the chicken thighs with salt and black pepper. Coat the chicken in the flour and tap off the excess.

2. Heat the oil in a large, non-stick frying pan over a medium heat. Fry the chicken, skin-side down first, until golden brown. Turn the chicken over to brown the other side and add the garlic, chilli and thyme.

3. Carefully pour away the excess oil and fat released from the chicken and return the pan to the heat. Add the white wine and allow it to reduce for a few minutes, then add 50ml water and the lemon zest and juice.

4. Cook for another 8–10 minutes on each side until the chicken is cooked all the way through before serving.

Per serving (2 chicken thighs each)					
Carbs	of which sugars	Protein	Fat	Fibre	Kcal
7.5g	1.4g	54g	58g	1.8g	817kcal

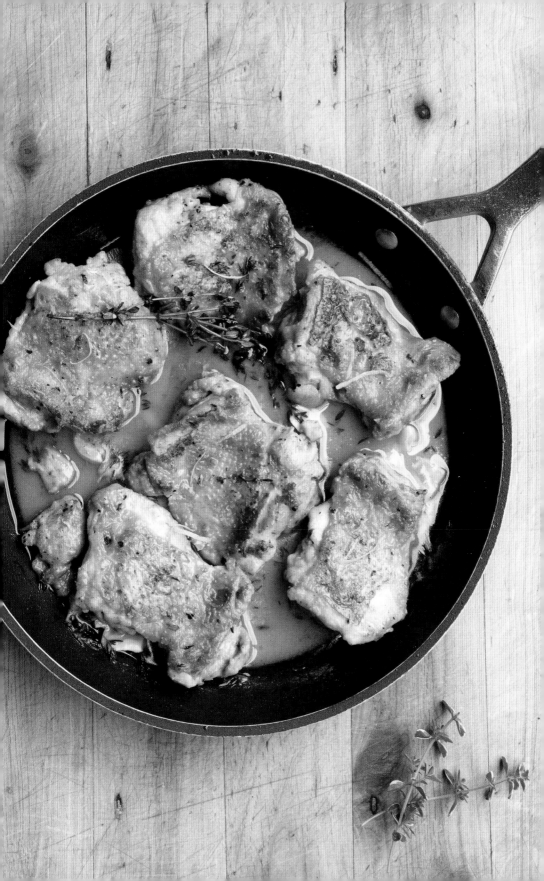

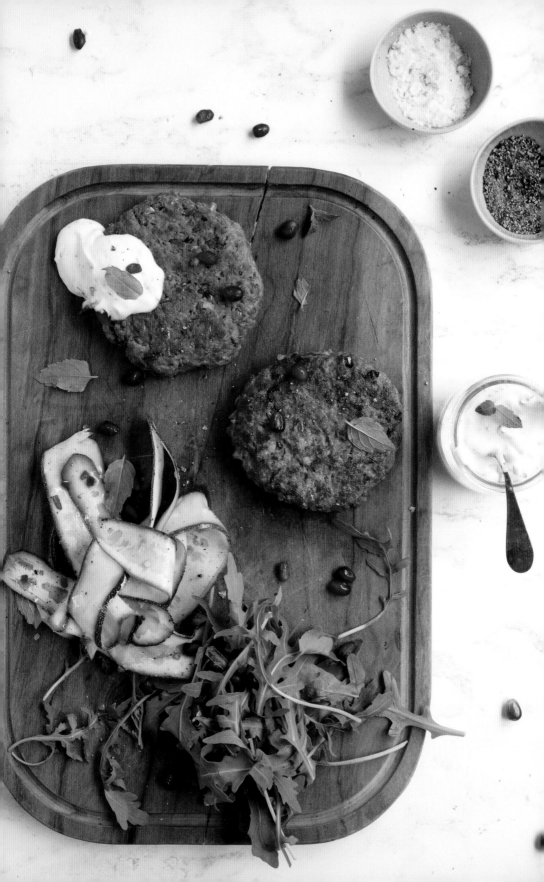

Harissa lamb burgers with courgette and pomegranate

Level	Prep time	Cook time	Days in fridge	Freeze
Intermediate	15 minutes	20 minutes	3	Yes

Serves 2

The harissa paste adds punchy flavour to the lamb here, making this a favourite one with kids.

3 tbsp olive oil
1 red onion, very finely diced
2 garlic cloves, grated
few sprigs fresh coriander, stalks and leaves separated and very finely chopped
2 tbsp harissa paste
400g minced lamb
salt and freshly ground black pepper

To serve
2 courgettes, cut with a peeler into ribbons
25g pomegranate seeds
100g natural Greek yoghurt
2 sprigs mint, leaves picked and chopped
handful of rocket

1. Place a small frying pan over a low-medium heat and add 1 tbsp of the oil. Add the red onion, garlic, coriander stalks and some salt and black pepper and fry gently for 8 minutes.

2. Add 1 tbsp of water to the onions towards the end of cooking, then stir in the harissa paste and remove from the heat. Leave to cool slightly.

3. Place the minced lamb into a bowl, add the onion mixture and work in using your hands.

4. Form the mixture into four burger patty shapes, flattening them so they are not too thick in the middle, and place in the fridge to rest for 5–10 minutes.

5. Meanwhile, toss the courgette ribbons with the pomegranate seeds and arrange onto plates.

6. Heat a large, non-stick frying pan over a medium heat and add the remaining 2 tbsp oil. Add the lamb burgers and cook for about 4 minutes on each side until they are cooked through. Rest the burgers in the pan for a few minutes covered with a lid.

7. Serve the burgers alongside the courgette and pomegranate mixture with dollops of yoghurt, the rocket and scattered with the coriander and mint leaves.

Per serving					
Carbs	of which sugars	Protein	Fat	Fibre	Kcal
13g	11g	49g	48g	5.4g	692kcal

Aubergine parmigiana v

Level	Prep time	Cook time	Days in fridge	Freeze
Moderate	15 minutes	60–75 minutes	5	Yes

Serves 2

Here is a wonderful veg-packed alternative to lasagne – and lower in carbs!

2 small aubergines, topped and tailed, cut lengthways into 1cm-thick slices
50ml olive oil
1 x 400g tin whole plum tomatoes
100g mozzarella, cut into very thin slices
30g Parmesan cheese (or vegetarian hard cheese alternative), grated
few sprigs of basil, leaves picked
salt

1. Preheat the oven to 220°C fan/240°C/gas mark 9 and line a baking tray with baking paper.

2. Brush the aubergine slices with the olive oil and season lightly and evenly with salt on both sides. Spread out on the lined baking tray and roast in the oven for 12–15 minutes or until lightly browned. Remove from the oven and turn the heat down to 180°C fan/200°C/gas mark 6.

3. Pour a quarter of the tin of tomatoes into an ovenproof dish measuring approximately 15 x 15cm and roughly chop/break them up with a spoon. Lay over a quarter of the aubergine slices. Top with a quarter of the mozzarella, Parmesan and basil leaves. Repeat this layering process three more times, finishing with a layer of the two cheeses.

4. Bake in the oven for 45–60 minutes until browned on top and bubbling. Serve.

Per serving					
Carbs	of which sugars	Protein	Fat	Fibre	Kcal
12g	9.7g	19g	39g	6.6g	488kcal

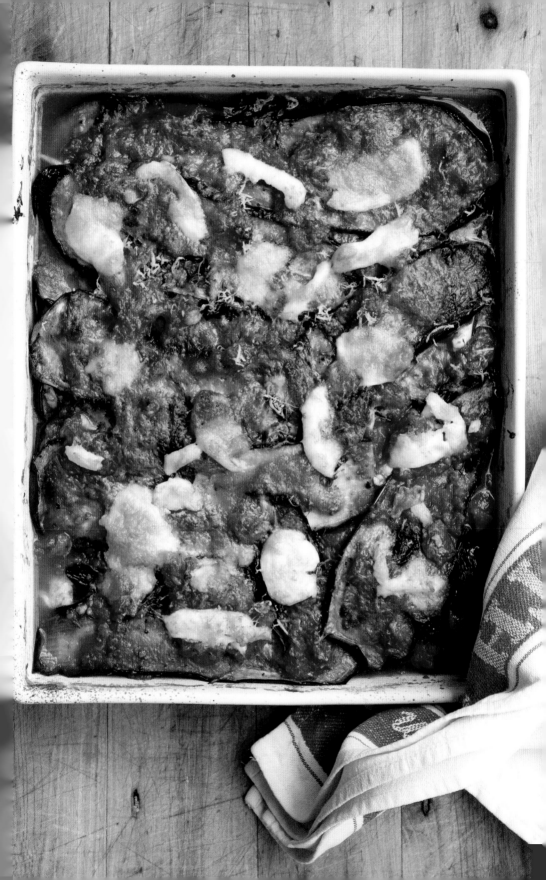

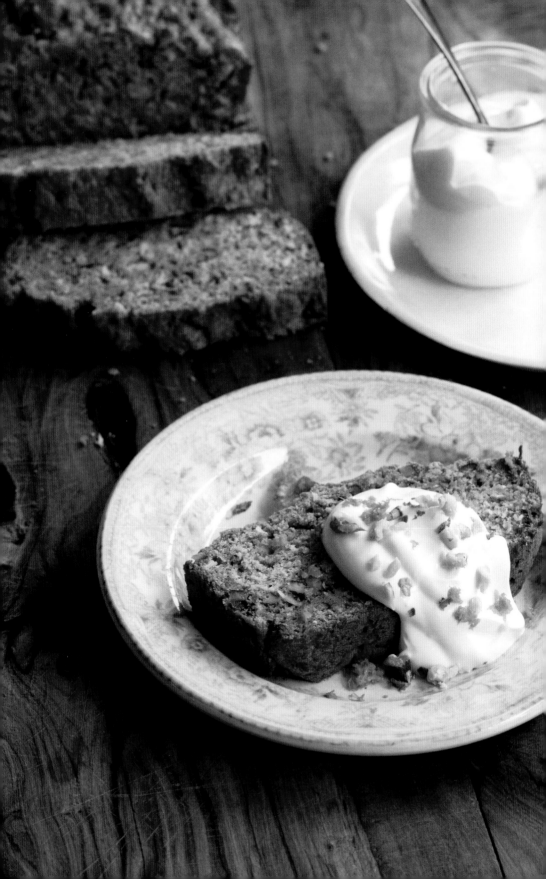

Carrot cake v

Level	Prep time	Cook time	Days in fridge	Freeze
Moderate	20 minutes	50–60 minutes	3	Yes

Makes 10 slices

We love this recipe. If you cannot find wholemeal self-raising flour you can use plain wholemeal flour and add 1½ tsp baking powder.

75g coconut oil, melted and cooled (or 100g unsalted butter, melted and cooled)
50g desiccated coconut (unsweetened)
100g unsweetened Greek yoghurt
2 free-range eggs
1 large ripe banana, peeled and mashed
2 tsp orange extract (optional)
185g wholemeal self-raising flour
½ tsp salt
½ tsp bicarbonate of soda
200g carrots, peeled and grated
50g walnuts or pecan nuts, broken into small pieces, plus extra to serve (optional)

To serve
100g unsweetened Greek yoghurt
grated zest of 1 orange

1. Preheat the oven to 180°C fan/200°C/gas mark 6.

2. Brush a 900g loaf tin (21.5 x 11cm) with a little of the melted coconut oil (or melted butter) and line the base with a strip of non-stick baking paper.

3. Put the remaining melted coconut oil (or butter), desiccated coconut, yoghurt, eggs, banana and orange extract (if using) in a mixing bowl. Mix together using a hand-held electric whisk or a large metal spoon. Set aside.

4. Sift the flour into a separate large bowl and add the bran from the sieve to the same bowl. Mix in the salt, baking powder (if needed) and bicarbonate of soda.

5. Gently fold the flour mixture into the wet ingredients with a large metal spoon. Add the carrots and nuts and fold again to combine, taking care not to overmix.

6. Tip into the prepared loaf tin and bake in the oven for 50–60 minutes or until a skewer inserted into the middle comes out clean.

7. Remove from the oven and leave to cool in the tin for 20 minutes. Run a knife around the edge and remove from the tin, then leave to cool completely on a wire rack.

8. Slice and serve with dollops of Greek yoghurt, grated orange zest and extra chopped nuts, if you like.

Per serving (1 slice)					
Carbs	of which sugars	Protein	Fat	Fibre	Kcal
17.5g	4.6g	7g	15.5g	2.6g	240kcal

Peanut butter and banana ice cream v

Level	Prep time	Days in freezer	Freeze
Easy	10 minutes	28	Yes

Serves 2

The texture of this is amazing – it is hard to believe it's not a cream-based ice cream and it also looks the same. Most of the sugar content in this recipe comes from the bananas; if you use slightly greener bananas, then the sugar content will be lower. You could also add a pinch of cinnamon to help regulate your blood sugar. When you have some bananas at home that are getting too brown, peel and chop them up and freeze in bags to use in recipes like this or in smoothies. If you are lactose intolerant, then just omit the yoghurt and milk and it will taste just as good!

You can buy ready-roasted peanuts or just use raw unsalted peanuts – place on a baking tray and roast in preheated to 180°C fan/200°C/gas mark 6 for 25 minutes, stirring at least twice.

3 ripe bananas, peeled and frozen
2 tbsp raw peanuts, roasted
1 vanilla pod, split and seeds scraped out
2 tbsp Greek yoghurt
3 tbsp full-fat milk

To serve
2 tbsp unsweetened peanut butter
2 tbsp roasted peanuts
25g melted dark chocolate (90% cocoa solids)
a little extra sliced fresh banana

1. Place the frozen peeled bananas and roasted peanuts in a high-speed blender and blitz until smooth and creamy.

2. Add the vanilla seeds, yoghurt and milk and blitz again to combine.

3. If you like soft-serve ice cream, then serve immediately in two bowls, each topped with peanut butter, roasted peanuts, melted dark chocolate and extra sliced banana. Delicious!

4. If you like it firmer, freeze in a shallow airtight container for 1 hour until set, but remove from the freezer 5 minutes before serving as above.

Per serving (including serving suggestion)

Carbs	of which sugars	Protein	Fat	Fibre	Kcal
40g	33g	18g	26g	6.1g	479kcal

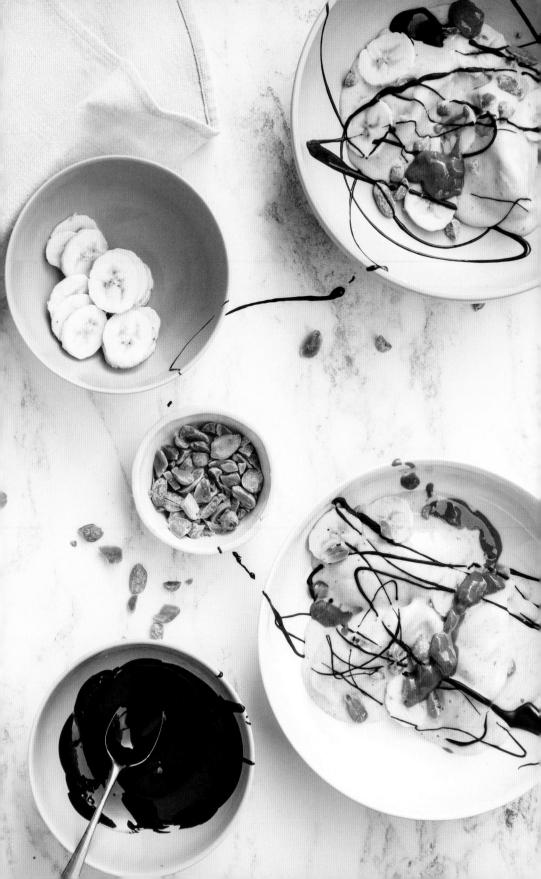

LOW
SUGAR
FOR LIFE

Well done on completing the challenge! You may have had a few hiccups along the way, but that is life.

Remember, at the beginning we asked you to complete a scorecard questionnaire? It is time to see what progress you have made by filling out the scorecard again, on the page opposite. Have you noticed any difference in your energy levels, your sleep or skin?

I hope you have discovered that you do not need sugar as a reward, and that there are lots of healthier and happier ways of rewarding yourself and your family instead. For me, when I forget and choose a rich dessert at a restaurant, I notice that I feel really lethargic and bloated within twenty minutes. I then remember that I don't need to finish a meal with something sweet and ask my wife to remind me not to order dessert or, if I am still hungry, to go for the cheese board. The last item eaten in a meal has the biggest effect on the teeth (Geddes 1994). So why not make it teeth friendly!

If you keep up the low sugar lifestyle, over time, you will notice a decrease in your dental bills and the dental team will remark on the health of your mouth. Remember dental disease is entirely preventable, so why suffer?

Hopefully, like me, you have started to have an appreciation for cooking and enjoying mixing flavours without just relying on sugar. Cooking from scratch is not only cheaper but much more fun too.

Beyond the 14 days

So, what happens now? This is not supposed to be just another fad diet, but a plan to give you the knowledge and skills you need to incorporate a new way of eating into your daily life. Your dietary changes need to be tailored to you and your family's lifestyle in order to keep it up long-term. There will be an element of long-term behavioural change necessary, as we discussed, regarding how you reward yourself with things other than sugar.

We recommend slowly introducing selected foods that you may have missed, one at a time, while listening to your body. We do not suggest just going back to your old diet after all your hard work. It is OK to have sugar in moderation, as long as it is part of a balanced diet and you know you are eating it! You may find that your old favourite sweet treats do not taste as good as you remember. I have patients who used to drink Diet Coke daily and then, having taken the challenge, they have found it tastes abhorrently sweet and don't go back to it.

Eating out

One of the biggest issues can be eating out, because you cannot see or control what goes into the food. Here are some tips that might help:

- Some cuisines are easier than others – good-quality Japanese or Italian restaurants often offer fresher, healthier dishes.
- Look at the menu online before booking a restaurant – why make your life difficult if a menu is limited? Plenty of restaurants offer healthier choices and it is improving all the time.
- Often, most of the sugar is in the sauces/dressings, so ask for your sauce on the side and then you can control how much you add.
- At the cinema, you could make and bring your own popcorn with coconut oil and cinnamon.

The 14-Day Sugar Challenge
Questionnaire

Circle a number for each question

DATE					

DENTAL	Yes			No	
I saw my dentist in the last year					
I have no cavities/fillings					
My gums do not bleed when I brush					

SLEEP	Agree				Disagree
I sleep well at night	1	2	3	4	5
I wake feeling refreshed	1	2	3	4	5

MOOD	Agree				Disagree
I feel confident and happy	1	2	3	4	5

ENERGY	Agree				Disagree
I do not frequently feel tired	1	2	3	4	5
My energy does not slump in the day	1	2	3	4	5

WEIGHT	Agree				Disagree
I am happy with my weight	1	2	3	4	5

FOOD	Agree				Disagree
I enjoy my meals	1	2	3	4	5
I do not crave sweet or savoury foods	1	2	3	4	5
I am motivated to cook	1	2	3	4	5

HEALTH
Please add any concerns/issues such as joints, allergies, digestion, etc.

All of our charts are available to print online at **www.rewardsproject.org** if you prefer not to write in this beautiful book.

Celebrations and cake

I love afternoon tea and cake. It is fine to have the occasional piece of cake but be aware that cake may taste much sweeter than you remember it after the challenge. In my house, we often bake using 25% of the recommended sugar in the recipes and it still works out great. Sugar rather than artificial sweeteners is needed in most baking recipes to give texture and the browning effect, so we don't advise using artificial sweeteners instead.

My friend Lou Walker has carried out some research into the office cake culture and I want to share some of her findings with you. She found that the popularity of the office cake culture is not so much for the cake itself, but more so due to the social effect of getting colleagues together during the working day. Most offices found that they were having cake too frequently, and that they would actually be happier having cake just once per month. Lou also found it was best to keep the cake/biscuits out of sight until cake time. At Bow Lane, all cakes and biscuits are now kept in a cake tin. This tends to stop the casual passer-by who actually doesn't want a slice of cake but finds it hard to resist when it is lying in the open! Offices should also offer fruit or nuts as an alternative to cake. The team could consider bringing other things back from holiday/business trips rather than food each time. Almost one-quarter of people surveyed found it hard to refuse cake if everyone else was eating it and then nearly two-thirds regretted eating it straight after. I would suggest discussing with the people in your office if and when they actually want cake, and how else they would like to celebrate their birthdays and special occasions. Actually, just going ahead and buying a cake without thinking is not in everyone's best interests.

You may have found that your body functions better without alcohol and this challenge has helped you realise that. You also could have used it to cut down. So why do we drink? Some people feel social pressure to drink alcohol so they fit in. As we have discussed (see page 47), most alcohol contains sugar, but some has a worse effect on your body than others.

What to do if you relapse?

If you do go off target, do not beat yourself up about it. Remember exactly how your body is feeling right now. One way of flushing that sugar out of you is to drink two big glasses of water and go out in the fresh air, do some exercise. Then reflect on what you can learn from this? Was it driven by a particular event or emotion?

Getting additional help and support

Your dental care professionals can help you, or you may want to discuss matters in more depth with a dietitian. Our Kick Sugar Facebook community is a good place to look for support and encouragement from others who have also been through the challenge.

Pass on the challenge

If you know anyone else who would enjoy rediscovering their full range of taste, please pass on the challenge to them. We find the biggest change happens when the whole family gets involved. The money goes towards the Charity, Rewards Project. Take a look here to see other ways you can become involved: **www.rewardsproject.org**

My final reward for you is a healthier version of yourself.

How to get your workplace involved

A great way to get your workplace involved in the challenge is to ask them to sign our pledge to create a sugar-free workplace for two weeks. Not everyone needs to be involved in the full challenge, but it is important that they respect your efforts by not bringing in or consuming sugar-laden foods during those two weeks. Encourage your colleagues to complete the questionnaire in this book before and after the two weeks, so they too can monitor the positive effects on their health. At Bow Lane Dental, we provided our team with healthy snacks and lunches during the two week period. Perhaps you can ask your workplace to do the same? Then all you need to think about is your own breakfasts and dinners. See an example of the pledge overleaf or download it from our website.

FALSE BELIEFS

• IT IS IMPOSSIBLE TO MAINTAIN LOW SUGAR FOR LIFE
It's absolutely possible to reduce and keep to a low amount of sugar in your diet. Once you know where to look for it and how to create great tasting food without it, you can ensure that you are eating well. You can train your body to not miss sugar at all.

TOP TIPS

1) Be fussier. There is a world of difference between a proper homemade cake and one produced in a factory, even if the homemade cake does include some sugar. Have a small piece, savour and enjoy!
2) Keep cake and sugary foods out of sight! If they are visible most people will eat them.
3) Step up your exercise to boost your metabolism and also improve your insulin sensitivity. Then the occasional treats will be less damaging.
4) If your place of work or study is a sugar haven – with chocolates on the side or frequent cake sharing – consider introducing your friends and colleagues to the 14-day sugar challenge and find alternative ways to celebrate.
5) Longer term, you may like to reintroduce the odd treat – OCCASIONALLY! Think special occasions and holidays…

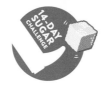

DATE: _ _ _ _ _ _ _ _
_ _ _ _ _ _ _ _ **WILL BE A SUGAR-FREE ZONE FOR TWO WEEKS WHETHER TAKING PART OR NOT**

During my 14-Day Sugar Challenge, I pledge to...
✔ Complete an anonymous questionnaire before and after my Challenge.
✔ Give feedback at the end of the Challenge.
✔ I would like free lunches for ten days.

NAME	TAKING PART? YES/NO	SIGNATURE

All of our charts are available to print online at **www.rewardsproject.org** if you prefer not to write in this beautiful book.

INDEX

W

Y

References

All nutritional analysis:
www.nutritics.com

If you want to find out how best to reward you and your family, visit
www.rewardsproject.org

Join our Kick Sugar Facebook community for help with kicking sugar for life

WITH THANKS TO...

This cookbook is a result of some amazing talented individuals who care about the health and wellbeing of our society. Jenny Phillips, a passionate CNHC registered Nutritional Therapist and author of *Eat to Outsmart Cancer*. Jenny helped me to better understand the nutritional impact of sugar upon the body and to co-write two of the chapters in this book. Having spent time with my friend and chef, Giancarlo Caldesi, I knew food can be both tasty and nutritious. Without his advice, his recipes, his kitchen and his sons Giorgio and Flavio, there would be no book (and a huge pile of washing-up!). Giancarlo's wife Katie, with an impressive portfolio of 14 cookbooks to her name, helped me to understand how to put the book together into a format that would work.

The Caldesis introduced me to Clare Gray, who is not only a registered dietitian, but also a chef and food stylist. She helped cook and prepare the recipes to make them look irresistible in the photographs. Charlotte Simpkins helped me test, tweak and develop these delicious recipes, not only to be nutritious, but also easy to prepare and cook. Rebecca Fennell is the wizard behind the camera, who turned my idea into the beautiful recipe photos you see here. Thank you also to Jenny Dack for her inspired illustrations and to Matt Inwood for shaping all of the above onto page so effectively. Editor Alice Sambrook was the best second pair of eyes an author could wish for. A third and final pair of eyes came via the careful proofreading of Anne Sheasby.

I have to thank my team at Bow Lane Dental Group for being the first people to do the 14-day challenge and support me throughout this journey.

Finally, my wife, Alison, who inspired the idea by her continuous frustrations with the unhealthy snacks/lunches/rewards on offer to our children in their daily life. Also, Harry, Kate and Emily for being expert tasters and giving me honest feedback on the recipes!